Books

INTUITIVE EATING
FOR TEENS

*The Teenagers Guide To Stop Dieting, Overcome Eating
Disorders, Emotional and Binge Eating*

LOOK AND FEEL GREAT WITH ANTI-DIET,
HEALTHY RECIPES FOR NATURAL WEIGHT LOSS

Amber Netting

DISCLAIMER

The recipes and information in this book are provided for educational purposes only. Please always consult a licensed professional before making changes to your lifestyle or diet. The author and publisher shall have neither liability nor responsibility to anyone with respect to any loss or damage caused or alleged to be caused directly or indirectly by the information contained in this book. All trademarks and brands within this book are for clarifying purposes only and are owned by the owners themselves, not affiliated with this document.

Images from shutterstock.com

CONTENTS

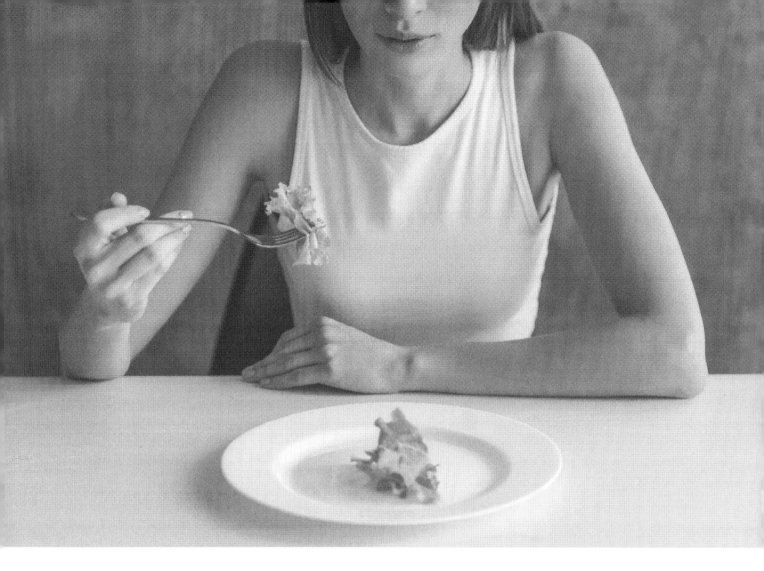

INTRODUCTION

Being a teenager isn't easy in our time of strict beauty standards when everyone can be made to feel ashamed of or judged for any little difference that doesn't meet those standards. And our weight isn't an exception to this, especially among young people. Being under pressure millions of teenagers suffer from eating disorders every day while trying to meet society's preferences and they don't even realize how harmful it can be to their health. Is there any way to help them?

I believe there is! And this book is about finding a solution in intuitive eating. It's a perfect eating practice for people who want to feel comfortable with their body and enjoy food at the same time, and it's also may be an answer for teens. Just listen to your body carefully, and you will be able to please it with maximum benefits for you. I want to warn you that it won't be easy at the beginning. Intuitive eating is not just about understanding your body's needs, but also about liberating yourself from worrying about your appearance–a lot of psychological work. So, I'm here to help you!

If you are a teen who struggles with your weight, then I'm glad that you found this book. With all my heart I hope I will help you to find a way to be in harmony with your body, so you can enjoy your life without any psychological and physical damage because of your look. I'm sure you are beautiful.

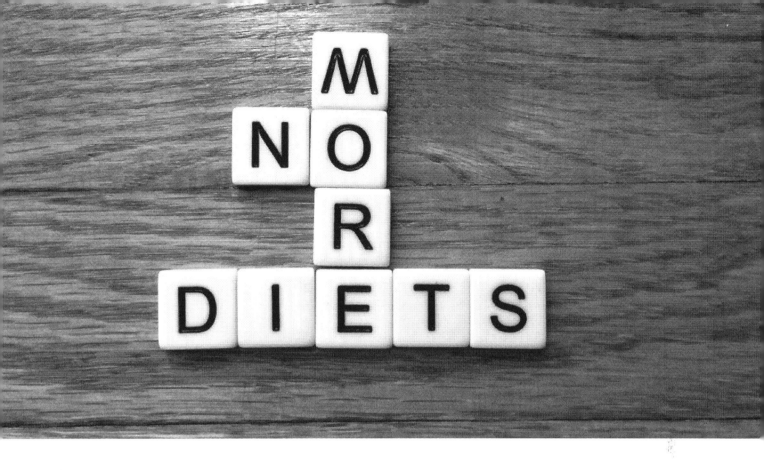

CHAPTER 1. BUILDING A HEALTHY RELATIONSHIP WITH FOOD

STARTING INTUITIVE EATING

1. START RIGHT NOW.

The intuitive eating principles can be implemented at your next meal or snack. Since it's about tuning in to yourself and being free from diet–y rules, there is no official start date.

While diets always begin tomorrow, intuitive eating can start right now. Days are not chalked up as successful or not depending on whether you do "good enough" intuitive eating. Intuitive eating is the antithesis of perfectionist thinking, all–or–nothing. Everything is an opportunity to learn, a chance to check in with yourself.

2. CHECK IN WITH YOUR HUNGER.

This is one of intuitive eating's most well–known tenets: eat when you are hungry, stop when you're full. That is where too many people stop. And so, intuitive eating becomes the hungry–full diet. Assessing your hunger level is an important piece of intuitive eating but it's just one part of the whole.

So, you want to check in with your stomach and look for a gnawing or empty feeling that tells you that you're hungry.

3. CHOOSE FOODS YOU ARE HUNGRY FOR.

Once you have determined your level of hunger, check with yourself what you would like to eat. Do your best to match what you want to eat and what you decide to eat.

Food is meant to be pleasant–and not just fuel. The entire act of eating is a life–enhancing experience. But if you see food as mere fuel and choose foods strictly by their nutritional components, you're missing out. And ironically, even when you're physically full, you're more likely to overeat or even binge.

Satisfaction eating is just as important as nutrition eating. A lack of satisfaction with your food choices easily leads to post–meal pantry–surfing. You can fill your stomach with food that you think you should eat, absolutely. But if you weren't hungry for that, you'll still feel unsatisfied–no matter how big the meal.

4. CHALLENGE DIET RULES.

After you check in to see if you're hungry, and what you're hungry for, negative thoughts are likely to pop up: "It's bad for me," "It's going to go right to my thighs," "It's toxic." Where did those messages originate from? Parents, teachers, coaches, friends, social media, etc.? Moralizing food is everywhere! And sadly, it all too often fires back. Food tastes far better without a side order of "I shouldn't eat this."

LINK BETWEEN BODY GROWTH AND EATING

As you grow older, you can start making your own choices about a lot of things that matter to you the most. You can choose your own clothes, your own music, and your friends. You may also be ready to take your own body and health decisions.

A great place to start is making healthy choices about what you are eating and drinking, how much sleep you are getting, and how active you are. Feed your developing body by making better food decisions as a teenager today and as you continue to grow into your 20's.

The teenage years are a time of rapid growth, which is why a healthy balanced diet is important. If you're a teenager, eating well–balanced meals is important, rather than having too many snacks that are high in fat, sugar, or salt.

Here are some tips:

TIP #1: GET OVER THE IDEA OF FOOD MAGIC
For good health, there are no magic foods to eat. Teens need to eat foods like vegetables, fruits, whole grains, protein foods, and dairy foods that are free of fat or low in fat. Choose foods with protein, such as unsalted nuts, beans, lean meats, and fish.

Whole grains that supply fiber can give you a feeling of fullness and provide you with key nutrients. Choose whole grains for half of your grains. Eat whole–wheat breads, pasta, and brown rice rather than white bread, corn, or other processed grains. Also, if you need to "fill-up" select vegetables and fruit.

TIP #2: KEEP WATER HANDY
Water is a better choice than many other drinks. Keep a bottle of water in your bag and on your desk to relieve your thirst. Avoid soda, fruit beverages, and sports and energy beverages. These are sweetened with sugar, and have few nutrients.

TIP #3: BUILD A LIST OF FAVORITES
Looks more like green apples than red apples? Ask your family food shopper to purchase quick–to–eat foods such as mini–carrots, apples, oranges, low–fat cheese slices or yogurt for the fridge.

TIP #4: START COOKING OFTEN
Get over hunger by cooking your own meals and snacks. Learn how to make vegetable omelets, bean quesadillas or a spaghetti pan. Prepare your own food so you can make meals and snacks healthier. Frozen microwave pizzas don't qualify as home cooking.

Different individuals require different quantities of calories to be active or to maintain a healthy weight. The number of calories you need depends on whether you are male or female, how old you are, whether you are still developing and how active you are, which may not be the same every day.

STOP DIETING

Teens really should be careful with dieting. Extreme diet can cause problems if you are not having the right nutrient types and quantities. But eating healthy meals and snacks and exercising will help you lose weight and encourage normal development.

Everyone needs enough calories to keep their bodies running smoothly. Any diet where you are not eating enough calories and vital nutrients can be detrimental to you. Heavy low–fat diets may be bad for you, too. Everybody requires some fat in their diet and no one can eat a diet that is fully free of fat. Approximately 30 per cent of calories should come from fat.

Don't go for food limiting diets. A diet that says nothing about carbohydrates — like bread or pasta — or asks you just to eat fruit is unhealthy. You will not be receiving the vitamins and minerals that you need. And while at first you can lose weight, those diets usually don't work long–term.

Eating a variety of nutritious foods is the optimal way to eat.

ENJOY FOOD AGAIN

It seems rather hard to have a healthy relationship with food in our diet–obsessed, restriction–focused society let alone a love affair with eating.

Many people worry that eating will lead to terrifying consequences. That they are going to eat everything in sight, and won't be able to control themselves. And many are just used to seeing food as the enemy, as the very thing that stands in the way of their goals for weight–loss or faultless figures.

And the very idea that we can enjoy food is not just scary, but also strange. It seems novel given the cultural climate we're in, where food is vilified and categorized into good and bad. Where people scorn their cravings and hunger signals.

There are many ways to make healthy choices and enjoy your meals. Try these ideas to add healthy eating enjoyment:

- Enjoying your meal should consist of choosing a variety of healthy foods and flavors you like

- Culture and food traditions can help in a great way to make your meal enjoyable
- There are a lot of ways to enjoy your meals on a budget
- There is no right way to enjoy your food; no matter what your lifestyle is, you can enjoy your food.

To find new foods to enjoy, try a variety of different healthy foods. It can appeal to a sense of wonder and even adventure to try new foods.

Part of enjoying your food can be in the surrounding atmosphere. The setting around you can help make the meal times more satisfying. Creating a positive eating environment can include:

- Meals with others
- Making your dining area appealing
- Turning some of your favorite background music on

Changing your relationship with food isn't that simple. But this is a good first step in starting to enjoy food, getting curious about what you like and don't like (not based on what some diet says) and learning to nourish yourself.

WARNING:

Reflections in this mirror may be distorted by socially constructed ideas of 'beauty'

CHAPTER 2. APPEARANCE AND FOOD: TEEN'S REALITIES

WORK WITH YOUR COMPLEXES

Most of us are ready to handle the evident physical changes of growing up. Yet before, during, and after puberty, the body also goes through certain changes — and often those changes may be very different from those we expect to happen. For example, both girls and guys can experience growing in unusual areas, like the butt or the belly. Or maybe they grow taller and skinnier.

We become more aware of our looks right around the time our bodies begin to change. This could make physical changes difficult to deal with emotionally. Adjusting to a changing body, though, is more than just how it looks. Many teens base their self–image on how they feel and how their bodies act. So, how can you help yourself to adjust emotionally and physically, without developing a lot of complexes?

Here are a few suggestions.

BEWARE — DON'T COMPARE IT!

It's natural to look at the comparison of our friends. But this isn't a good idea. Comparing ourselves with others is problematic because we all develop differently and at different times. If you're going through a growth spurt early, you might feel too tall. Yet your friend might think that he or she is too small. It's usually the hardest thing for people to develop first or last.

Comparing ourselves with the celebrities and models is also a bad idea. In real life, people don't look like the limited types of bodies that appear in the media. (Models often don't really look like that either: Many of those "perfect" bodies got that way through photo editing, not nature.) Ads sell fantasy, not reality.

TREAT YOUR BODY WELL.

Making educated food and exercise choices is a part of developing your own mind and life. Eating and exercising healthily can also give you some control over how your body turns out. What's more, exercise is a mood booster. If you feel sad or confused about your changing body, it may help you to go for a walk, throw a Frisbee with your friends, or play with your dog.

BEFRIEND YOUR BODY.

Feeling like you no longer know your body? Just like a growing and evolving friendship, it takes time to keep in touch with our bodies. Like friends, our bodies can sometimes let us down, but it's possible to bounce back with some work and understanding.

Just as we know the secrets of our friends, we know things of our own bodies that other people do not know. You may think, for example, that your stomach sticks out because in the mirror you spend hours concentrating on that. But the truth is that other people will not notice it the way you do.

What people notice is how you project your self-centered feelings. If you think you're too tall, if you slump over and try to look smaller, it'll be more noticeable. Hiding behind your hair can cover the zit on your cheek if you're self-conscious about your pimples — but you'll look awkward and uncomfortable.

It can help to work on having good posture as your body changes and walk with a sense of confidence. You'll probably become more confident after doing this for a while, too.

You can't really do much about your height or development, but you can focus on the things you really like about yourself. It's perhaps your curly hair, or the dimple that you get when you smile. Perhaps it's that you're a very thoughtful person or that you're good at making people laugh.

In the end, when you think of the people that you care about the most in your life, what they look like probably has very little to do with how much you like them.

DEALING WITH EMOTIONS

The teen years come with all sorts of changes, so it's normal to feel up and down emotionally. If a person struggles with additional weight, this may add to those emotions.

Not everyone who is overweight is concerned or upset about that, of course. Many of us know people who are overweight, confident and happy — and thin, fit people who are insecure. But since people often feel pressure to look a certain way, adolescents with weight problems may feel bad about themselves.

You may feel frustrated, angry, or upset when you're overweight. The first step in dealing with difficult emotions is being aware of them.

Recognizing emotions takes practice. They can sometimes be so sudden and powerful that it is difficult to sort out exactly what you feel. The best way to do that is to pause and pay attention

for a moment when you first feel upset. Try to name what feelings you feel without judging yourself. Say to yourself, "I feel angry" (or frustrated, or sad.)

If you're upset, but you don't know exactly why, it can help to talk to someone you trust, like a family member, a close friend, or a therapist. Speaking about things can also help people figure out how to deal with their feelings.

If it's challenging to talk about your feelings or you think people don't understand, keep a journal, draw or paint, or do anything else that helps you sort through difficult emotions. The more time you take to explore your feelings, the more ability you get to cope with emotions as they arise. That can make finding solutions to the problems easier.

ACCEPTING BODY NATURE

Have you ever wanted to change something about your body? If yes, then you are not alone. Lots of people feel unhappy with some of their appearance. But if you're stuck on what you don't like it can really bring your self-esteem down. Do you want your best look and feel?

ACCEPT YOUR BODY

No one is and can be perfect. Everyone wants to be liked, respected, and accepted just as themselves. This also holds true for every BODY! See the way your body is. Be less critical. Be more friendly.

Don't body-shame yourself. It hurts your self-esteem when you make harsh comments about your own body. That's true, whether you think it yourself, or say it out loud. It hurts as much as having someone else say it. Be friendly. Respect yourself even if there are things you need to work on.

Build improved habits. Have you got used to putting down your body? Build a good one in its place, to break that bad habit. Say what you like and don't say what you don't. Hold on until it's a habit.

LIKE YOUR BODY

Find what you like about your looks. You may like your hair, your face or your hands. Your shape, shoulders, or legs? The eyes, or the smile? Say what you like and why. If you get stuck, think about the way you look to your good friends. Accept those things. Know there is plenty to like about you. Let that feel good for yourself.

TAKE CARE OF YOUR BODY

Eat good food. Learn what food is right for you, and how much is right. Take your time eating. Taste your food really well. Enjoy this. Eating right helps you to look the best you can. It's giving you the energy that you need. And it boosts your image of your body. You feel good about yourself when you treat your body correctly.

Sleep well. Learn how much you need to sleep for your age. Get yourself to bed on time. Turn off screens ahead of bedtime so you can sleep well.

Be active every single day. Your body needs movement to be healthy, fit, and strong. Playing a sport can be active. You can run, walk, work, do yoga, swim, dance, etc. Pick the things you like.

Make the most of the fun you can have.

AVOCADO AND POACHED EGG TOAST

SERVINGS: 1   PREP TIME: 5 min.   COOK TIME: 5 min.

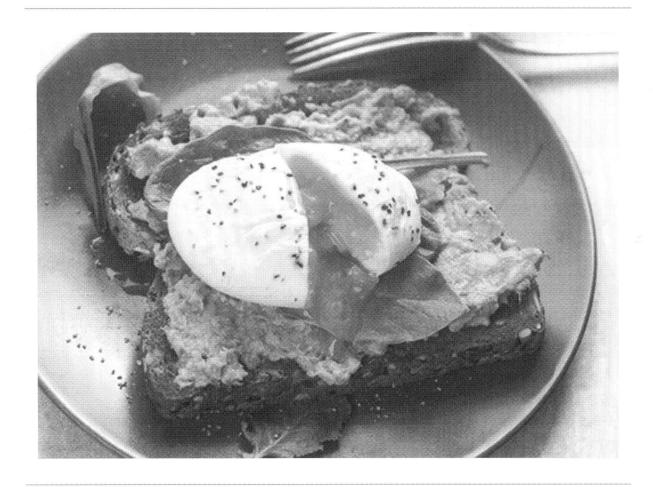

CARBS–30 g   FAT–20 g   PROTEIN–23 g   CALORIES–393

INGREDIENTS

- *2 fresh eggs*
- *⅓ avocado*
- *2 slices whole grain bread*
- *¼ cup fresh spinach leaves*
- *Salt and pepper for topping*
- *Fresh herbs (parsley, thyme, or basil) for topping*

DIRECTIONS

1. Add enough water to a pot to cover the eggs and bring to a boil.

2. Drop two metal outer rims of mason jar lids into the pot and make sure they lie flat on the bottom. When it boils, turn off the heat and crack the eggs into each rim. Cover and poach for 5 minutes.

3. Meanwhile, toast your bread and smash avocado on each piece of toast.

4. When the eggs are done, lift them out of the water using a spatula. Pull the rim off of the eggs.

5. Put the poached eggs on top of the toast. Sprinkle with salt, pepper, and fresh herbs.

6. Serve with fresh spinach leaves or other green leaves.

CLASSIC CAPRESE FRITTATA

SERVINGS: 3 PREP TIME: 5 min. COOK TIME: 25 min.

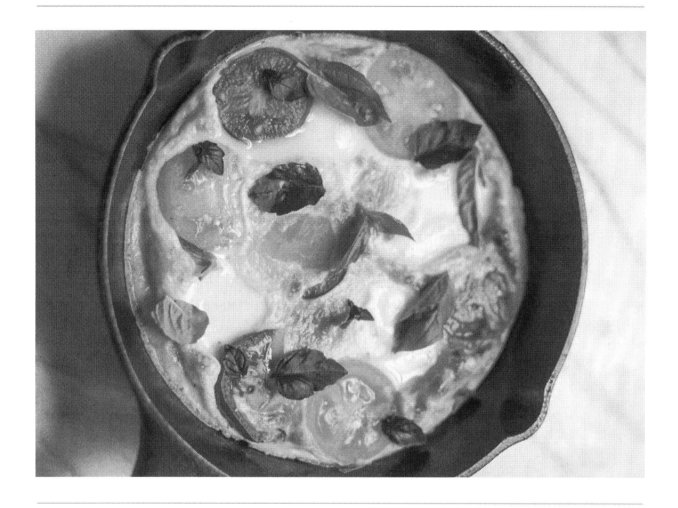

CARBS–10 g   FAT–33 g   PROTEIN–31 g   CALORIES–460

INGREDIENTS

- 6 large eggs
- ¼ cup any milk
- 2 garlic cloves, minced
- ¼ tsp sea salt
- Black pepper, to taste
- Extra–virgin olive oil, for drizzling
- 1 shallot, chopped
- 2 cups cherry tomatoes, halved
- ¾ cup mozzarella balls, halved
- ½ cup basil, sliced

DIRECTIONS

1. Preheat the oven to 400°F.
2. Whisk the eggs, milk, garlic, and salt until combined. Set aside.
3. Heat ½ Tbsp of olive oil in a cast–iron skillet over a medium heat.
4. Add the shallot, salt, and pepper and cook for 5 minutes.
5. Add the tomatoes, half the basil, stir, then add the egg mixture and shake the pan to distribute.
6. Add the mozzarella and bake for 15–20 minutes or until the eggs set.
7. Top with the rest of the basil and serve.

HEALTHY BREAKFAST SMOOTHIES

SERVINGS: 1   PREP TIME: 5 min.   COOK TIME: 5 min.

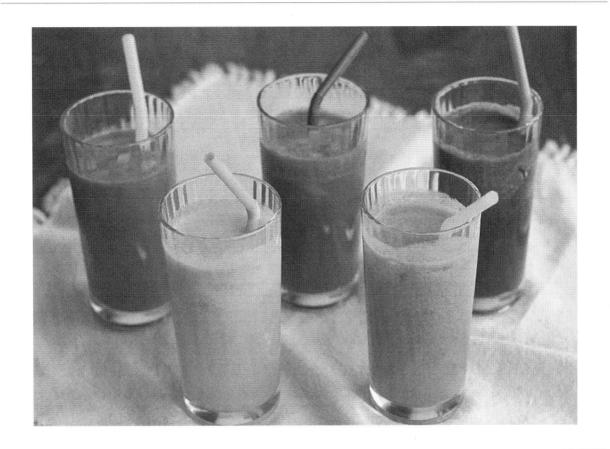

CARBS–34 g   FAT–3 g   PROTEIN–6 g   CALORIES–190

INGREDIENTS

ADD TO EACH SMOOTHIE:
- ⅓–¾ cup Almond milk
- A few pieces of ice

FOR THE PEACH SMOOTHIE:
- 1 peach, sliced
- ½ cup raspberries
- ⅓ Tbsp almond butter
- ½ banana

FOR THE STRAWBERRY SMOOTHIE:
- ½ cup strawberries, sliced
- ¼ cup dried goji berries
- ½ banana

FOR THE BLUEBERRY SMOOTHIE:
- ⅓ cup tart cherries
- ⅓ cup blueberries
- ⅓–1 Tbsp raw cacao powder
- ½ banana

FOR THE MANGO SMOOTHIE:
- ½ large mango slices
- 1 peach, sliced
- 1 tsp maca powder
- ½ banana

FOR THE SPINACH MANGO SMOOTHIE:
- ½ large mango slices
- 1 handful of fresh spinach
- 1–2 tsp matcha
- ½ banana

DIRECTIONS

1. To prepare your smoothies ahead of time, add the fruit to containers and then put into the freezer until you're ready to blend.
2. Blend the ice and almond milk for 30 seconds.
3. Then, add in the fruit and blend for 30 seconds–1 minute more until smooth.
4. Pour into a glass and enjoy.

FRENCH TOAST WITH FRESH BERRIES

SERVINGS: 4   PREP TIME: 5 min.   COOK TIME: 15 min.

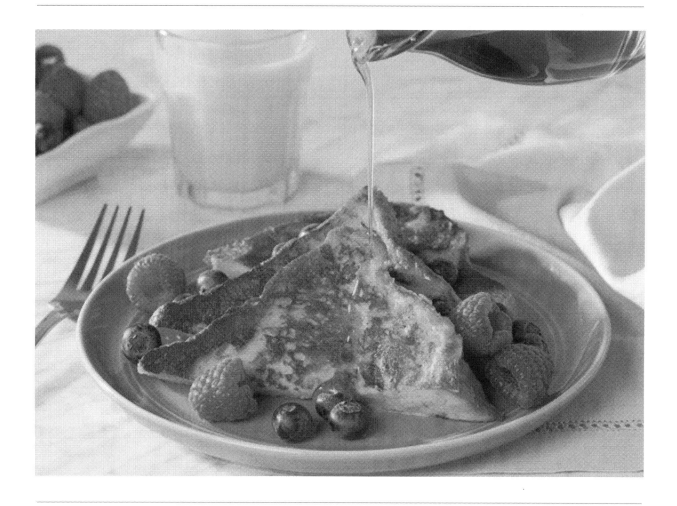

CARBS–19 g   FAT–5 g   PROTEIN–7 g   CALORIES–156

INGREDIENTS

FOR THE TOAST:
- 4 eggs
- 1 cup any milk
- 1 tsp cinnamon
- ¼ tsp cardamom
- Pinch of sea salt
- 8 1–inch slices challah bread or preferred bread
- Coconut oil, for brushing

FOR SERVING:
- 1 cup raspberries
- 1 cup blueberries
- Maple syrup, to taste

DIRECTIONS

1. Whisk the eggs, milk, cardamom, cinnamon, and salt in a bowl. Dip the bread into the mixture and place on a large plate or tray.
2. Heat a skillet over a medium heat and brush with oil. Put in the bread slices and cook for 2 minutes per side until golden brown. Turn the heat to low to cook thoroughly without burning (if needed).
3. Serve with maple syrup and berries.

FRUIT AND GRAIN YOGURT BOWLS

SERVINGS: 1   PREP TIME: 5 min.   COOK TIME: 5 min.

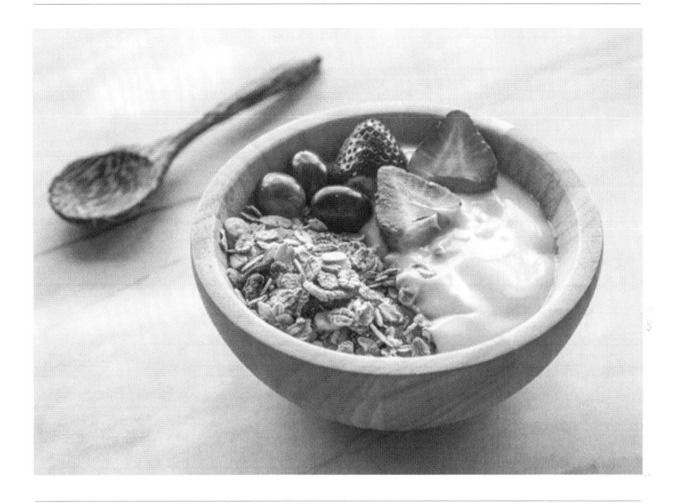

CARBS–11 g   FAT–5 g   PROTEIN–5 g   CALORIES–102

INGREDIENTS

- *1 cup Greek yogurt*
- *1 cup prepared grain of choice*
- *1 cup fresh strawberries and cherries*
- *Honey or maple syrup, to taste*

DIRECTIONS

1. Spoon the yogurt into a bowl.
2. Top it with the prepared grain and fresh berries.
3. Add honey or maple syrup, and enjoy!

CLOUD EGGS

SERVINGS: 4   PREP TIME: 5 min.   COOK TIME: 15 min.

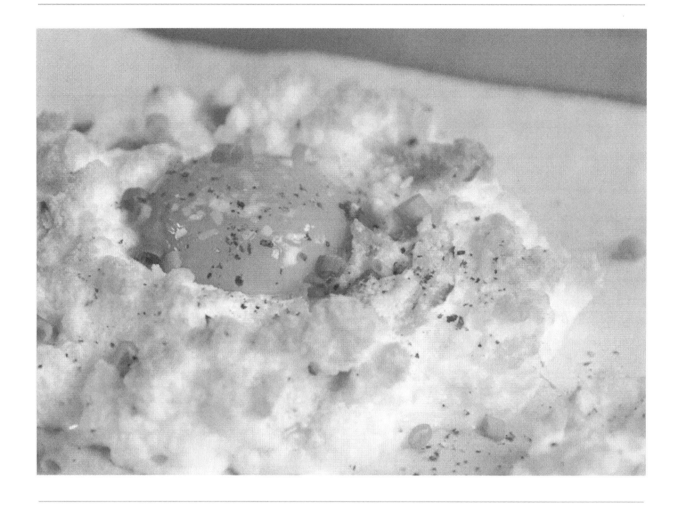

CARBS–1 g   FAT–9 g   PROTEIN–14 g   CALORIES–139

INGREDIENTS

- *8 large eggs*
- *1 cup freshly grated Parmesan*
- *½ lb. deli ham, chopped*
- *Kosher salt*
- *Freshly ground black pepper*
- *Freshly chopped chives, for garnish*

DIRECTIONS

1. Preheat the oven to 450°F and oil a baking sheet by greasing it with cooking spray.
2. Separate the egg whites and yolks, putting the yolks into a small bowl and the whites into a large bowl. Using a whisk, beat the egg whites for 3 minutes until stiff peaks form. Carefully fold in the cheese and ham, then add salt and pepper.
3. Using a spoon, make 8 mounds of egg whites on a greased baking sheet and form nests by indenting the centers. Bake for 3 minutes until lightly golden.
4. Gently spoon egg yolk into the center of each nest. Bake for 3 more minutes until the yolks set.
5. Take out of the oven and sprinkle with chives before serving.

GREEK YOGURT PANCAKES

SERVINGS: 3–4   PREP TIME: 10 min.   COOK TIME: 15 min.

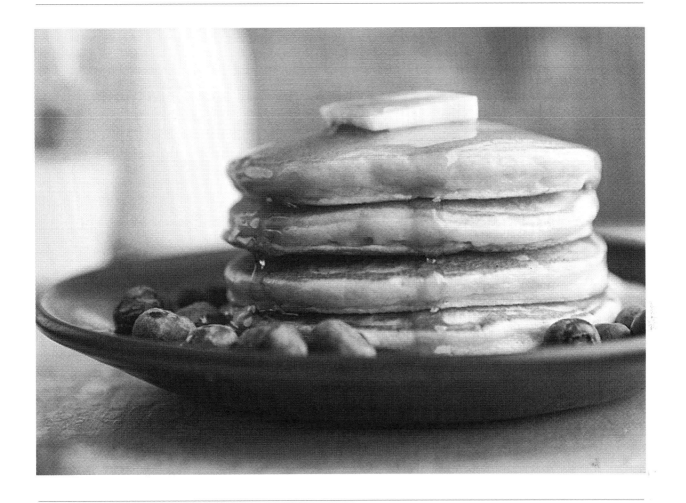

CARBS–47 g   FAT–2 g   PROTEIN–22 g   CALORIES–296

INGREDIENTS

- *1 cup flour*
- *2 eggs*
- *1 Tbsp baking powder*
- *1⅔ cups Greek yogurt*
- *1 cup blueberries, for serving*
- *3–4 butter slices, for serving*

DIRECTIONS

1. Whisk the baking powder and flour in a large bowl. In another bowl, whisk the eggs and yogurt, then fold it into the flour mixture to make a thick batter.
2. Pour it into the pan and cook for 1–2 minutes on each side over a medium–low heat, using a spoon to smooth out the batter into a ¼–inch thick pancake shape.
3. Cook until both sides are lightly golden. Repeat for the rest of the batter.
4. Serve the warm pancakes with fresh blueberries and top with maple syrup and a butter slice.

KALE FETA EGG TOAST

SERVINGS: 2   PREP TIME: 5 min.   COOK TIME: 20 min.

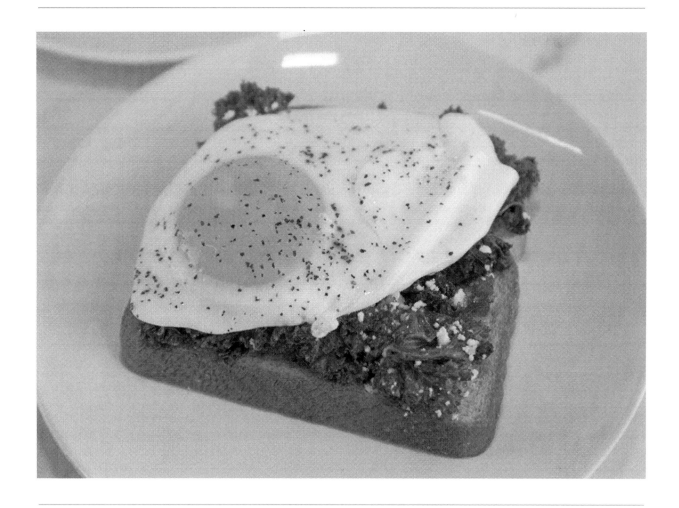

CARBS–2 g   FAT–7 g   PROTEIN–12 g   CALORIES–149

INGREDIENTS

- 2 slices bread of choice, toasted
- 3 tsp olive oil, divided
- 3 cups kale, chopped and stems removed
- 1 tsp minced garlic
- ⅛ tsp salt
- ⅛ tsp pepper
- 2 large eggs
- 2 ounces feta cheese, crumbled

DIRECTIONS

1. Heat 2 tsp of olive oil in a large skillet over a medium heat. Add the kale and cook, occasionally stirring for 5 minutes. Add the garlic, salt, and pepper. Stir and cook for 1 more minute. Add in the cheese, cover, and remove from the heat.
2. Heat 1 tsp olive oil in another skillet over a medium heat. Crack in the eggs and season to taste. Cook for 1 minute or until the whites are nearly set. Cover the skillet, remove from heat, and leave for 3 minutes.
3. Arrange half of the kale on top of each piece of toast and top with a fried egg.

CHICKEN OMELET

SERVINGS: 1   PREP TIME: 10 min.   COOK TIME: 10 min.

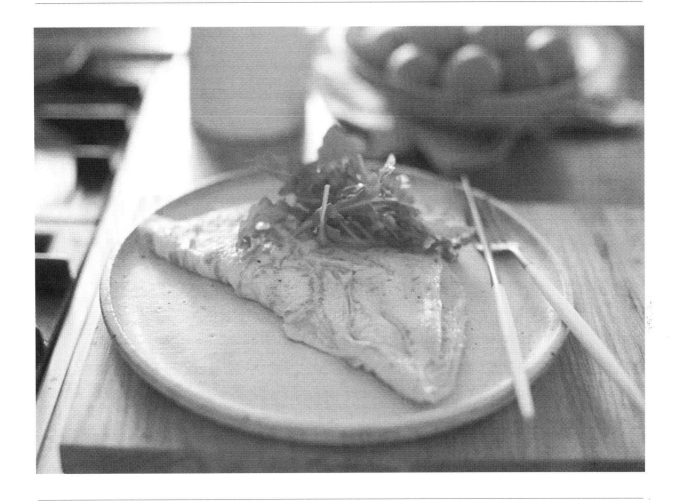

CARBS–22 g   FAT–8 g   PROTEIN–22 g   CALORIES–250

INGREDIENTS

- *4 eggs, beaten*
- *Salt and pepper, to taste*
- *1 tsp olive oil*
- *⅓ cup cooked, shredded chicken*
- *2 Tbsp shredded gruyere cheese*
- *¼ cup arugula, for serving*

DIRECTIONS

1. Whisk the eggs until well combined, then season with salt and pepper.
2. Heat 1 tsp of oil in a cast–iron skillet on a high heat.
3. Pour the eggs into the skillet and turn to low. Swirl the eggs to coat the bottom. Let it cook for 1–2 minutes.
4. Add the chicken and cheese to half of omelet. Cook for 30 more seconds.
5. Fold the other half over the filling. Cook for 1 minute or until the cheese has melted.
6. Serve with a few leaves of fresh arugula on top.

SWEET POTATO HASH

SERVINGS: 4   PREP TIME: 20 min.   COOK TIME: 30 min.

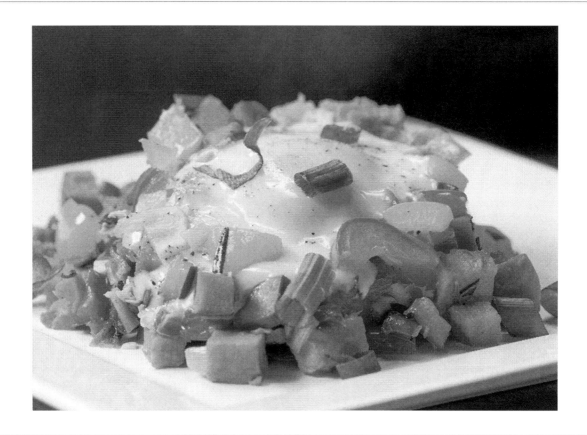

CARBS–27 g   FAT–21 g   PROTEIN–19 g   CALORIES–371

INGREDIENTS

- *3 strips bacon*
- *1 pound sweet potatoes washed, peeled, and cubed*
- *½ red pepper diced*
- *½ yellow onion diced*
- *½ tsp chili powder*
- *½ tsp cumin*
- *½ tsp paprika*
- *½ tsp dried oregano*
- *½ tsp garlic powder*
- *½ tsp salt + more to taste*
- *½ tsp black pepper*
- *1 cup shredded cheese of choice*
- *3–4 large eggs*
- *1 pinch scallions, for serving*

DIRECTIONS

1. Put the bacon in a cold cast iron skillet (oven–safe) in one layer over a medium heat.
2. Cook the bacon until crispy, then remove from the pan. Crumble it and set aside.
3. Add the potatoes to the same skillet and cook for 5 minutes until they start to soften.
4. Add in the red pepper, onion, and all seasonings. Cook for 7–10 minutes.
5. Preheat the oven to 400°F.
6. Once the vegetables are done, add the crumbled bacon and cheese. Stir well.
7. Form 3–4 shallow indents into the hash, using the back of a spoon.
8. Crack an egg into each indent.
9. Put in the oven and bake until the egg whites have set (10–15 minutes).
10. Sprinkle with chopped scallions before serving.

TERIYAKI CHICKEN VEGETABLES

SERVINGS: 4   PREP TIME: 10 min.   COOK TIME: 20 min.

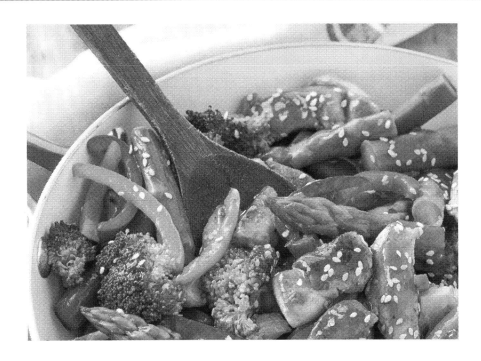

CARBS–21 g   FAT–8 g   PROTEIN–15 g   CALORIES–220

INGREDIENTS

FOR THE SAUCE:
- ¼ cup soy sauce
- ⅓ cup water
- 2 tsp minced garlic
- 1 tsp minced ginger
- 2 Tbsp honey
- 1 Tbsp brown sugar
- 2 tsp toasted sesame oil
- 1 Tbsp 1 tsp cornstarch

FOR THE STIR–FRY:
- 1¼ lbs. chicken breast cut, into 1–inch pieces
- 2 cups broccoli florets
- 1 red bell pepper, cut into1–inch pieces
- 1 yellow bell pepper, cut into1–inch pieces
- Salt and pepper to taste
- 1 Tbsp vegetable oil
- 1 Tbsp sesame seeds, toasted

DIRECTIONS

1. Heat 1 tsp of oil over a medium–high heat in a pan.
2. Add the broccoli and peppers, then sprinkle with salt and pepper. Cook for 4–5 minutes. Add 2 Tbsp of water and cook to evaporate it. When the vegetables are crisp and tender, remove from pan and set aside.
3. Wipe out the pan. Heat 2 tsp oil over a high heat in the pan.
4. Add half of the chicken to the pan and season it with salt and pepper. Cook for 3–4 minutes per side or more until completely cooked through. Transfer onto a plate and set aside. Repeat for the second half of the chicken.
5. Meanwhile, mix all of sauce components in a bowl.
6. Put the chicken and vegetables back into the pan. Pour in the sauce and cook for 2–3 more minutes over a medium–high heat.
7. Sprinkle with sesame seeds and serve.

CHICKEN AND SWEET POTATO BOWLS

SERVINGS: 3   PREP TIME: 10 min.   COOK TIME: 35 min.

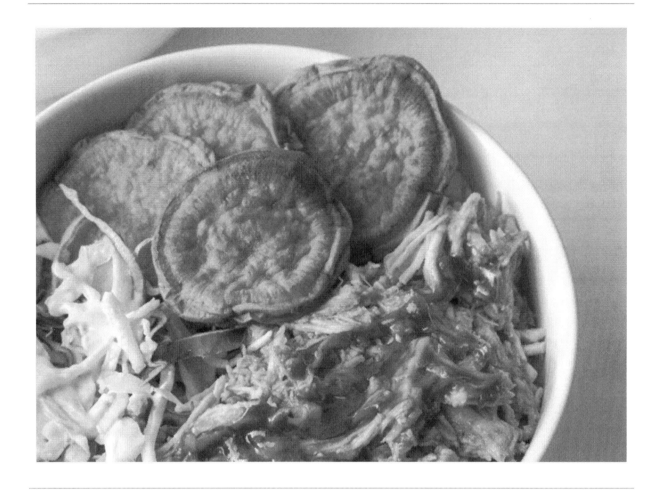

CARBS–53 g   FAT–13 g   PROTEIN–34 g   CALORIES–447

INGREDIENTS

- 2 medium sweet potatoes, sliced into rounds
- 1 large yellow onion, chopped
- 2 Tbsp olive oil, divided
- ½ tsp salt, divided
- ½ tsp garlic powder
- ½ tsp chipotle powder
- 1 lb. boneless, skinless chicken breasts
- ½ cup BBQ sauce, divided
- Salt, to taste

DIRECTIONS

1. Preheat the oven to 400°F.
2. Add the onion and sweet potatoes to a lined sheet pan. Sprinkle with 1 Tbsp of olive oil, ¼ tsp of salt, garlic, and chipotle powder and toss to combine well. Bake at 400°F for 20 minutes.
3. Toss the potatoes and move to one side of the pan. Add 1 Tbsp of oil and ¼ tsp of salt, and toss again. Add the chicken and brush with half of the sauce. Bake for 15–20 more minutes until the chicken is done.
4. Remove the breasts from the pan and shred, using two forks. Toss the chicken with the rest of the sauce.
5. Add the roasted potatoes, chicken, and garnish of your choice to the bowls and serve.

GREEK CHICKEN

SERVINGS: 4   PREP TIME: 40 min.   COOK TIME: 20 min.

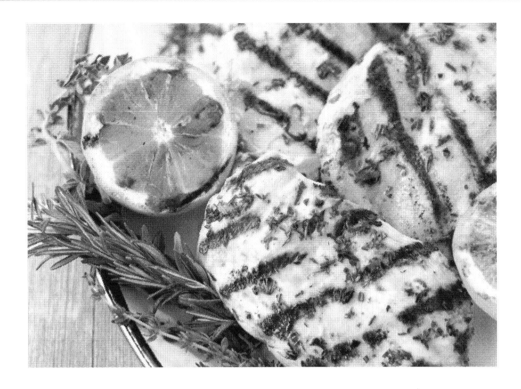

CARBS–12 g   FAT–14 g   PROTEIN–38 g   CALORIES–332

INGREDIENTS

FOR THE CHICKEN:
- Juice of 2 large lemons
- 2 Tbsp olive oil
- 4 Tbsp prepared spice mix
- 2 large boneless, skinless chicken breasts

FOR THE SPICE MIX:
- 1 tsp salt
- 2 tsp garlic powder
- 1 tsp onion powder
- 2 tsp dried basil
- 2 tsp dried oregano
- 2 tsp paprika
- 1 tsp black pepper
- 1 tsp dried rosemary, minced
- 1 tsp dried dill
- 1 tsp dried marjoram
- ½ tsp ground thyme
- ½ tsp ground nutmeg

FOR SERVING:
- 1 lemon, halved
- 3–4 fresh rosemary sprigs

DIRECTIONS

1. Mix all of the spices for the seasoning together. Set aside.
2. Divide each chicken breast into two even pieces. Rub the prepared spice blend all over the meat. Transfer into a plastic bag with the lemon juice and the olive oil. Leave to marinate for 30 minutes.
3. Preheat the grill pan over a medium–high heat. Grill the chicken for 8–10 minutes on each side. Check if it's done with a thermometer, it should be 165°F in the center. Take out of the grill and let it rest for 5 minutes before slicing.
4. Grill the lemon halves for 30 seconds–1 minute to give them nice grill stripes.
5. Serve the warm chicken with the grilled lemon and fresh rosemary sprigs.

STIR–FRY CHICKEN AND VEGETABLES

SERVINGS: 4   PREP TIME: 10 min.   COOK TIME: 15 min.

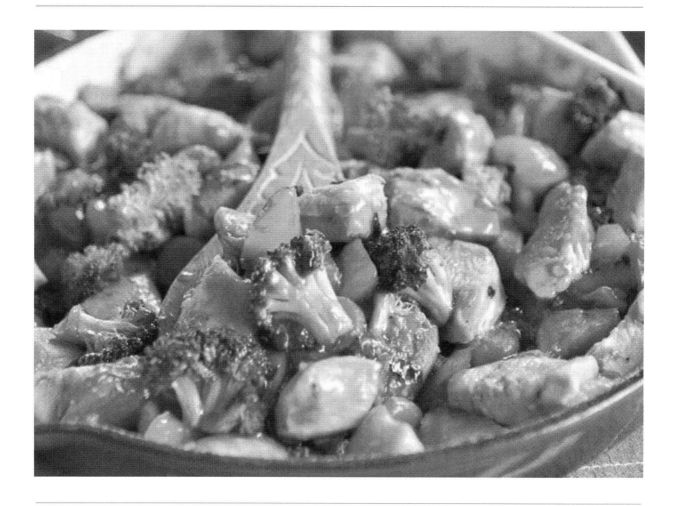

CARBS–32 g   FAT–9 g   PROTEIN–13 g   CALORIES–260

INGREDIENTS

- *2 Tbsp olive oil*
- *1 pound boneless, skinless chicken breasts, cut into pieces*
- *2 cups broccoli florets*
- *1 large zucchini cut into slices*
- *1 medium bell pepper, cut and sliced*
- *1 medium yellow onion, halved and sliced*
- *3–4 cloves garlic minced or crushed*
- *1 Tbsp Italian seasoning*
- *1 tsp salt*
- *⅓ tsp black pepper*

DIRECTIONS

1. Heat the oil in a large skillet over a medium–high heat.
2. Add the chicken, vegetables, garlic, and all of the seasoning. Cook for 8–10 minutes, stirring until the chicken is golden and completely cooked.
3. Serve with the garnish of your choice.

CHICKEN AND VEGETABLE RICE

SERVINGS: 4   PREP TIME: 5 min.   COOK TIME: 15 min.

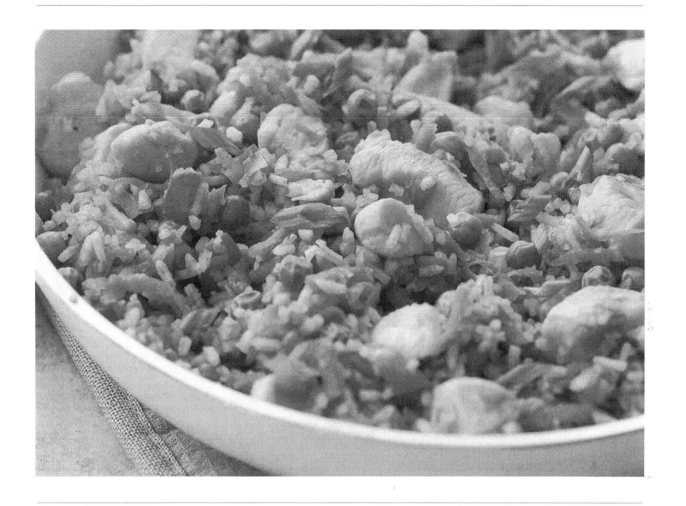

CARBS–64 g   FAT–25 g   PROTEIN–50 g   CALORIES–683

INGREDIENTS

- *3 Tbsp olive oil*
- *1 large sweet onion, diced*
- *1 medium red bell pepper, diced*
- *1 pound boneless skinless chicken breast, diced*
- *4 cups cooked rice*
- *1 cup peas*
- *3 cloves garlic, minced*
- *¼ cup water*
- *1 tsp paprika*
- *1 tsp cardamom*
- *Kosher salt, to taste*
- *Black pepper, to taste*
- *3 green onions, sliced into thin rounds*

DIRECTIONS

1. Add the oil and onions to a large skillet. Cook for 5 minutes over a medium–high heat until soft and translucent. Stir frequently.
2. Add the chicken and peppers, and cook for 5 minutes or until almost cooked through, stirring.
3. Add the garlic and cook for 1 more minute.
4. Add the broccoli, rice, water, and seasoning, stir to combine. Cover and cook for 5 more minutes.
5. Sprinkle with sliced green onions before serving.

TURKEY AND FRIED BELL PEPPERS

SERVINGS: 4   PREP TIME: 10 min.   COOK TIME: 10 min.

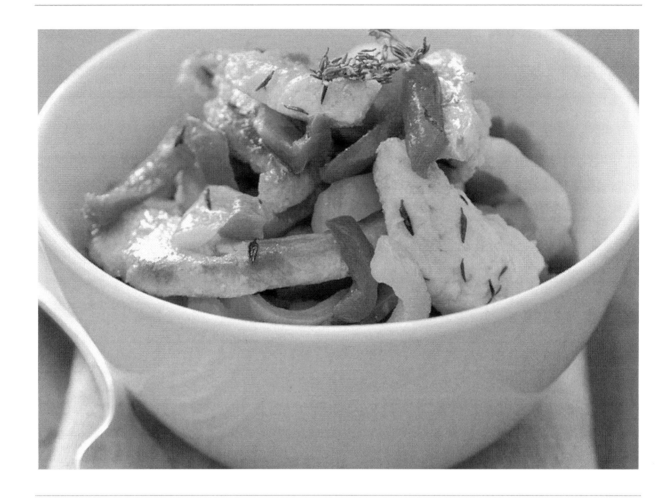

CARBS–11 g   FAT–8 g   PROTEIN–30 g   CALORIES–280

INGREDIENTS

- *1 pound turkey tenderloin, cut into steaks ¼–inch thick*
- *2 Tbsp extra–virgin olive oil, divided*
- *1 red bell pepper, cut into strips*
- *⅓ sweet onion, sliced*
- *1 tsp salt, divided*
- *1 yellow bell pepper, cut into strips*
- *⅓ tsp Italian seasoning*
- *¼ tsp ground black pepper*
- *1 14–ounce can crushed tomatoes*
- *1 pinch fresh dill, chopped*

DIRECTIONS

1. Season the turkey slices with ½ tsp of salt.
2. Heat 1 Tbsp oil over a medium–high heat in a large skillet.
3. Add half of the turkey and cook for 5 minutes until cooked through, stirring.
4. Put the turkey on a plate and cover with foil.
5. Heat 1 Tbsp of oil in the skillet over a medium heat and repeat with the rest of the turkey.
6. Add the onion, peppers, and the rest of the salt to the skillet, cover and cook for 5–7 minutes, removing lid occasionally to stir.
7. Open the lid, increase to a medium–high heat and sprinkle with seasoning. Cook for 20 seconds–1 minute, stirring often. Add the tomatoes and bring to a simmer.
8. Add the turkey and bring to a simmer again. Cook for 1–2 minutes on a low heat to warm the turkey.
9. Serve topped with dill.

CHICKEN SESAME NOODLES

SERVINGS: 4   PREP TIME: 10 min.   COOK TIME: 15 min.

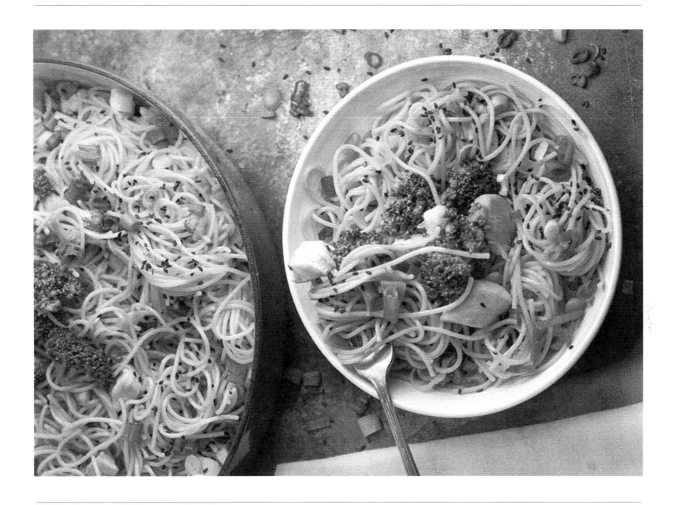

CARBS–54 g   FAT–16 g   PROTEIN–37 g   CALORIES–520

INGREDIENTS

- *½ lb. capellini pasta*
- *2 Tbsp olive oil*
- *2 cups broccoli florets*
- *1 lb. boneless, skinless chicken breasts, cut into strips*
- *½ cup toasted sesame dressing*
- *2 Tbsp soy sauce*
- *¼ tsp ground ginger*
- *¼ tsp garlic powder*

DIRECTIONS

1. Cook the pasta according to the package instructions, adding the broccoli to it for the last 3 min.
2. Meanwhile, heat the oil in a large non-stick skillet over a medium-high heat.
3. Add the chicken and cook for 6–8 minutes or more until cooked through, stirring occasionally.
4. Add in the soy sauce, sesame dressing, and spices. Cook for 1 more minute.
5. Drain the pasta and broccoli, then transfer to a large bowl. Add the chicken and stir well to combine.
6. Serve.

TACO WITH GROUND TURKEY

SERVINGS: 7   PREP TIME: 10 min.   COOK TIME: 15 min.

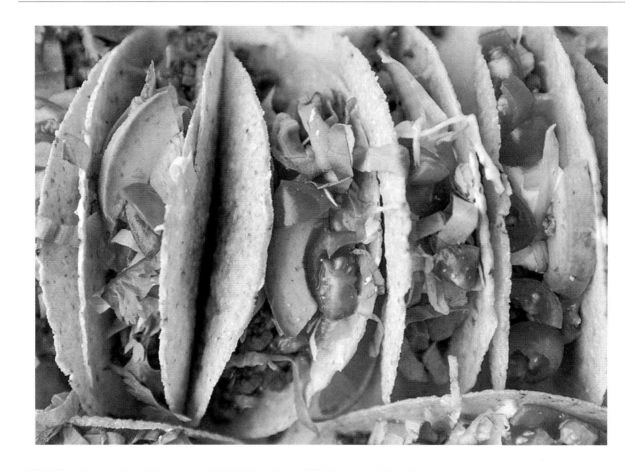

CARBS–6 g   FAT–5 g   PROTEIN–15 g   CALORIES–139

INGREDIENTS

- *1 tsp extra virgin olive oil*
- *1 onion, chopped*
- *2 jalapeño peppers, seeded and chopped*
- *2 cloves garlic, minced*
- *1 pound lean ground turkey*
- *2 tsp chili powder*
- *1 tsp cumin*
- *1 tsp garlic salt*
- *1 cup tomato sauce*
- *3 Tbsp tomato paste*
- *6–7 taco shells*

OPTIONAL TOPPINGS:
- *avocado slices, shredded cheese, diced tomato, fresh cilantro*

DIRECTIONS

1. Heat the oil in a skillet over a medium–high heat.
2. Add the onion and jalapenos; cook for 5 minutes, stirring frequently.
3. Add in the garlic cloves and cook for 1 minute, stirring. Transfer the onion mixture to a small bowl and set aside.
4. Add the turkey to the same skillet. Cook for 10 minutes, stirring until the turkey is cooked and no longer pink.
5. Add the cumin, chili powder, and garlic salt.
6. Add onion mixture, tomato sauce and paste and mix well. Reduce to a medium–low heat, stirring for 8 minutes until mixture starts to get thicker.
7. Serve in the taco shells with optional toppings.

CHICKEN NOODLE STIR-FRY

SERVINGS: 2 PREP TIME: 10 min. COOK TIME: 20 min.

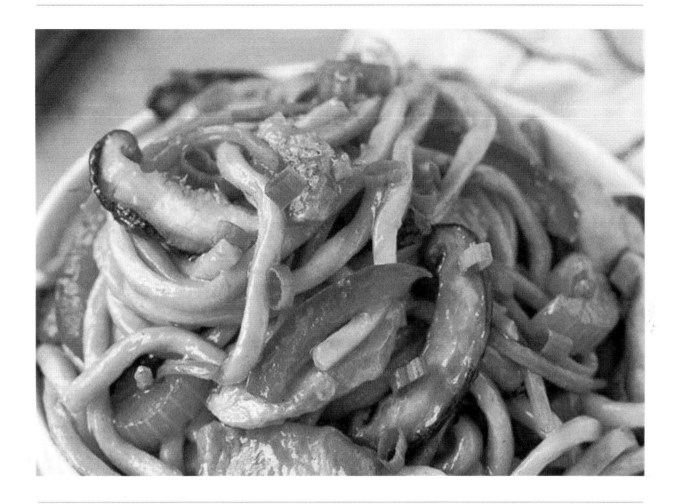

CARBS–20 g   FAT–2 g   PROTEIN–28 g   CALORIES–236

INGREDIENTS

- *2 nests dried egg noodles*
- *1 Tbsp olive oil*
- *2 chicken thighs, skinned, deboned and cubed*
- *1 garlic clove, finely sliced*
- *1½ cups broccoli florets*
- *2 Tbsp soy sauce*
- *1–inch ginger, peeled and finely chopped*
- *1 red pepper, cut into strips*
- *½ cup button mushrooms, sliced*
- *1 celery stalk, finely sliced*

DIRECTIONS

1. Cook the noodles according to instructions. Drain and toss with oil to avoid sticking.
2. Heat the oil in a pan and add the chicken. Cook over a high heat, stirring until golden.
3. Add the garlic and ginger. Cook for 30 seconds.
4. Add the vegetables and cook for 3–4 minutes, tossing. Check if meat is cooked through.
5. Pour in the soy sauce and add the noodles. Stir to combine.
6. Divide between two bowls and serve while hot.

MEDITERRANEAN TURKEY SKILLET

SERVINGS: 6   PREP TIME: 15 min.   COOK TIME: 25 min.

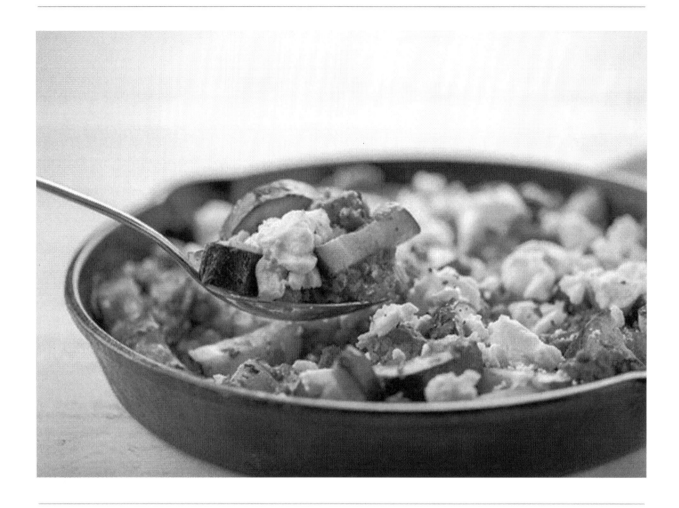

CARBS–20 g   FAT–10 g   PROTEIN–24 g   CALORIES–259

INGREDIENTS

- *1 Tbsp olive oil*
- *1 package lean ground turkey*
- *2 medium zucchinis, quartered and cut into ½–inch slices*
- *1 onion, chopped*
- *2 banana peppers, seeded and chopped*
- *3 garlic cloves, minced*
- *½ tsp dried oregano*
- *1 can black beans, rinsed and drained*
- *1 can tomatoes, undrained*
- *1 Tbsp balsamic vinegar*
- *½ tsp salt*

DIRECTIONS

1. Heat the oil over a medium–high heat in a large skillet.
2. Add the zucchini, turkey, peppers, onion, garlic, and oregano. Cook for 10–12 minutes or more to make sure the vegetables are tender, and the turkey is no longer pink. Break up the turkey into crumbles while stirring. Drain the liquids from the skillet.
3. Add in the rest of the ingredients and stir to combine. Cook for 3–4 minutes, stirring to heat through.
4. Serve hot and enjoy!

CHICKEN RAMEN

SERVINGS: 4   PREP TIME: 10 min.   COOK TIME: 20 min.

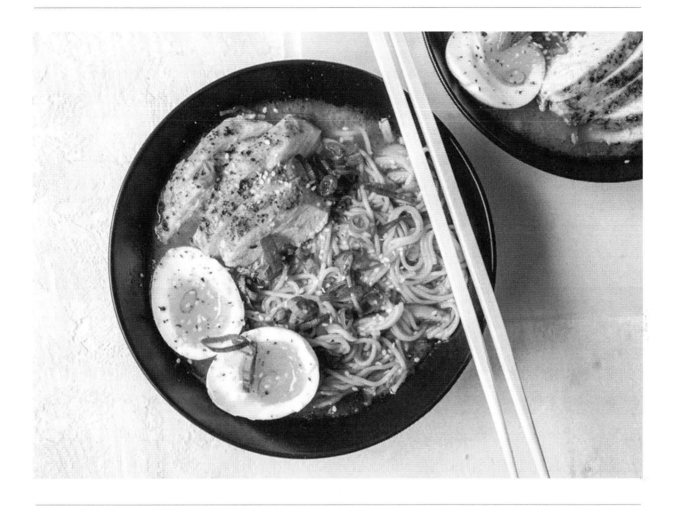

CARBS–38 g   FAT–6 g   PROTEIN–31 g   CALORIES–339

INGREDIENTS

- *2 eggs*
- *4 cups chicken broth, low sodium*
- *1½ tsp soy sauce, low sodium*
- *2 chicken breast fillets, boneless and skinless*
- *6–8 oz. ramen noodles*
- *1 cup cabbage, sliced*
- *1 cup carrots, shredded*
- *2 green onions, chopped*
- *Salt and pepper, to taste*

DIRECTIONS

1. Put the eggs with shells still on into a saucepan and cover them with water (1-inch). Let it boil, and take off the heat. Cover with a lid and leave for 7 minutes. Transfer to a bowl with ice. Set aside. You can hard boil the eggs if desired.
2. Meanwhile, add the chicken broth and soy sauce to another pot and bring to a boil. Add the breasts, and boil for 8–10 minutes until thoroughly cooked.
3. Remove the chicken from the broth and let them cool. Using two forks, shred the meat. Put the shredded chicken back into the pot.
4. Add the noodles. Cook for 3–5 minutes. Season with salt and pepper to taste.
5. Peel the eggs and cut them in half, set aside.
6. Turn off the heat. Add the cabbage and carrots. Serve immediately.
7. Garnish with egg halves and green onions.

CAJUN BEEF AND VEGETABLE RICE

SERVINGS: 4   PREP TIME: 10 min.   COOK TIME: 25 min.

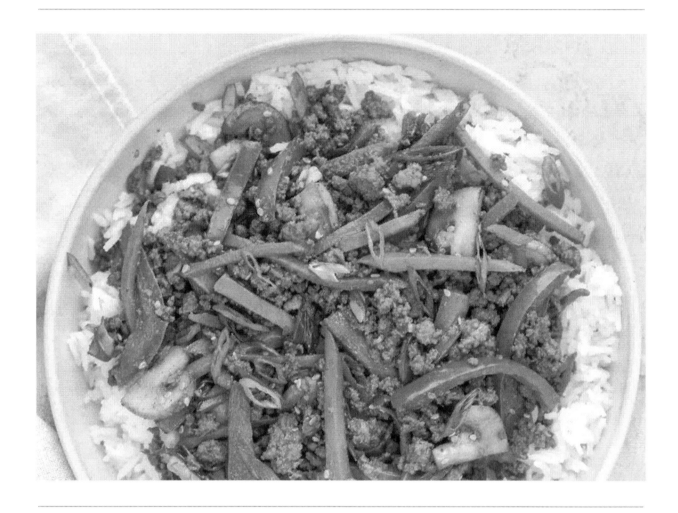

CARBS–53 g   FAT–12 g   PROTEIN–32 g   CALORIES–456

INGREDIENTS

- 1 Tbsp olive oil
- 500g 5% fat beef mince
- 1 celery stick, finely chopped
- 2 x 250g packs rice cooked
- 3 carrots, sliced into rounds
- 250 g mixed peppers, sliced
- 4 spring onions, sliced
- 2 tsp Cajun seasoning
- 1 tsp tomato puree

DIRECTIONS

1. Heat the oil in a large, shallow casserole dish over a medium heat. Add the celery, carrots, peppers, and white parts of the spring onions. Cook for 10 minutes until it starts to soften.
2. Add the mince and cook for 10 more minutes.
3. Add the seasoning and tomato puree, stir well. Add 4 Tbsp of water to the skillet and cook for 2–3 minutes.
4. Sprinkle with the chopped green parts of the spring onions and serve.

BEEF STIR-FRY

SERVINGS: 6   PREP TIME: 20 min.   COOK TIME: 15 min.

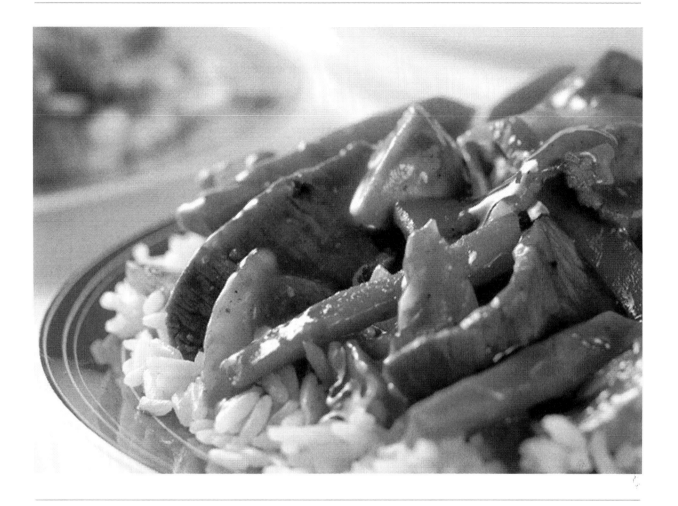

CARBS–10 g   FAT–16 g   PROTEIN–35 g   CALORIES–342

INGREDIENTS

FOR THE SAUCE:
- *4 Tbsp reduced-sodium soy sauce*
- *1 Tbsp rice vinegar*
- *1 Tbsp honey*
- *1 tsp cornstarch*

FOR THE STIR-FRY:
- *2 Tbsp vegetable oil, divided*
- *1½ lb. sirloin steak, cut into thin strips*
- *1 cup snow peas*
- *1 medium onion, sliced*
- *2 bell peppers, cut into thin strips*
- *1 Tbsp minced garlic*
- *1 Tbsp minced fresh ginger*
- *1 Tbsp sesame oil*
- *1 tsp sesame seeds, toasted*

DIRECTIONS

1. Mix all of the sauce components in a bowl and set aside.
2. Heat 1 Tbsp of oil in a skillet over a medium-high heat. Add the beef and fry for 2 minutes, until it's no longer raw. Transfer onto a plate.
3. Heat the rest of the oil in the same skillet.
4. Add the onions and peppers. Cook for 4–5 minutes until tender.
5. Add the garlic, ginger, and peas. Cook for 1–2 minutes, stirring.
6. Pour the sauce into the skillet and add the meat back in. Cook for 1 more minute, stirring.
7. Drizzle the beef with sesame oil and sprinkle with sesame seeds before serving.

GROUND BEEF WITH VEGETABLES

SERVINGS: 4   PREP TIME: 15 min.   COOK TIME: 20 min.

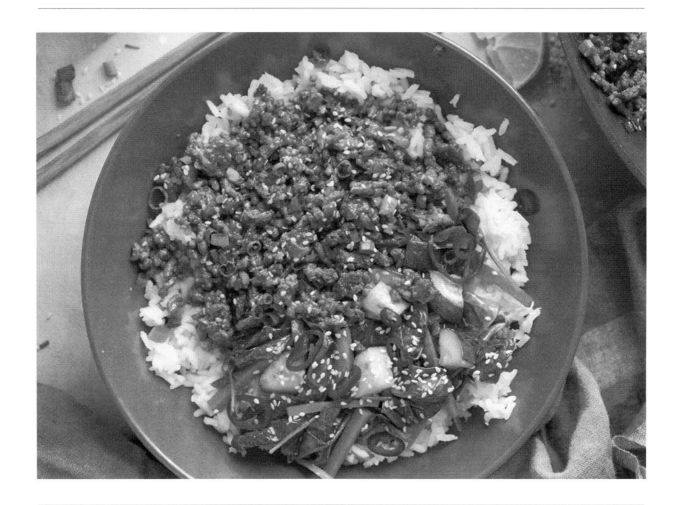

CARBS–17 g   FAT–10 g   PROTEIN–35 g   CALORIES–296

INGREDIENTS

- *3 cups mixed vegetables (red peppers, zucchinis, carrots, leafy greens)*
- *2 Tbsp water, more if needed*
- *¼ cup reduced sodium soy sauce*
- *2 Tbsp. brown sugar*
- *2 tsp sesame oil*
- *1 tsp Asian garlic chili paste*
- *2 garlic cloves, minced*
- *1 Tbsp ginger, minced*
- *1⅓ lbs. ground beef*
- *1 Tbsp sesame seeds, toasted*
- *¼ cup scallions, chopped*

DIRECTIONS

1. Heat a skillet over a medium–high heat. Add the vegetables and water. Cover and cook for 3–4 minutes until the veggies become tender–crisp. If they start to stick or burn, add more water. Remove from the pan and set aside.
2. Add the beef to the same pan. Cook for 8–10 minutes until it is cooked through, breaking it up.
3. Mix the brown sugar, soy sauce, chili paste, sesame oil, garlic, and ginger in a small bowl. Add to the beef and bring it to a simmer. Cook for 3–4 minutes.
4. Add the vegetables and sprinkle with chopped scallions and sesame seeds before serving.

ROAST BEEF

SERVINGS: 4   PREP TIME: 7 h.   COOK TIME: 20 min.

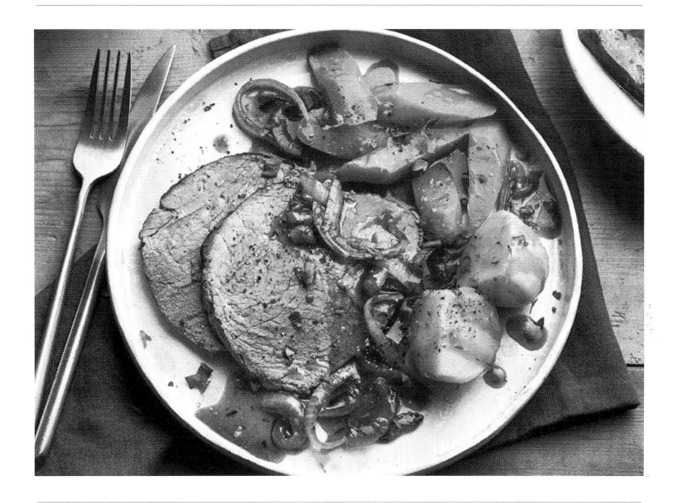

CARBS–25 g   FAT–18 g   PROTEIN–33 g   CALORIES–415

INGREDIENTS

- 600 g boneless beef chuck roast
- 600 g carrots, sliced
- 400 g potatoes, diced
- 2 onions, halved
- 4 stalks celery, thinly sliced
- 400 g can diced tomatoes
- 1 cup reduced–salt chicken stock
- 1 Tbsp fresh ginger, chopped
- 2 tsp dried oregano
- 1 tsp ground coriander

SPECIAL EQUIPMENT:
- Slow cooker

DIRECTIONS

1. Set the slow cooker to low.
2. Layer the carrots and potatoes on the bottom, then place the meat on top. Pour in the stock and add the tomatoes and spices.
3. Cover with the lid and set to 7 hours on low.
4. Take out the meat and leave it to rest covered on a carving board.
5. Put the carrots on a serving plate and cover with tin foil.
6. Pour the juices into a saucepan and cook for 5–10 minutes over a high heat to reduce slightly and make it thicker.
7. Slice the meat and serve with the potatoes, carrots, and sauce.

ITALIAN BURRITOS

SERVINGS: 8   PREP TIME: 20 min.   COOK TIME: 20 min.

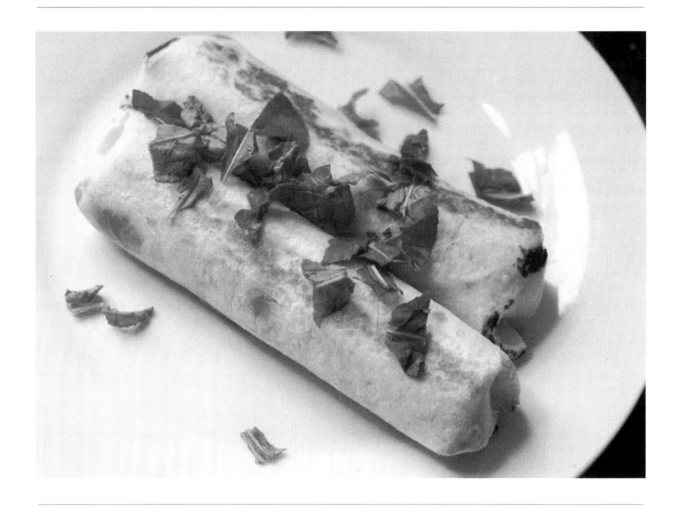

CARBS–26 g   FAT–10 g   PROTEIN–18 g   CALORIES–275

INGREDIENTS

- *1 pound lean ground beef (90% lean)*
- *1 cup marinara sauce*
- *½ cup shredded part–skim mozzarella cheese*
- *¼ cup grated Parmesan cheese*
- *¼ teaspoon garlic powder*
- *8 whole–wheat tortillas*
- *¼ cup chopped parsley, for serving*

DIRECTIONS

1. Preheat the oven to 375°F.
2. Add the beef to a large skillet and cook for 6–8 minutes over a medium heat or until it's no longer pink. While cooking, break it into crumbles. Drain the liquid and the add cheese, marinara sauce, and garlic powder.
3. Arrange ⅓ cup of filling in the middle of each tortilla. Fold the bottom and sides over the filling and roll it up.
4. Transfer onto a baking sheet coated with cooking spray.
5. Bake for 20 minutes until the bottoms are light brown.
6. Sprinkle with chopped parsley and serve.

COD WITH TOMATOES AND BASIL

SERVINGS: 4   PREP TIME: 10 min.   COOK TIME: 25 min.

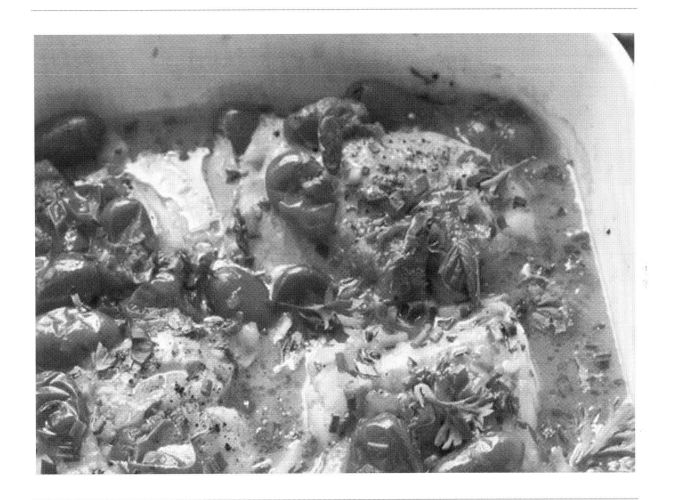

CARBS–5 g   FAT–11 g   PROTEIN–26 g   CALORIES–227

INGREDIENTS

- *3 Tbsp olive oil*
- *2 cups grape tomatoes*
- *1¼ lb. cod fillets 4–6 pieces 1–inch thick*
- *Salt, pepper and chili flakes to taste*
- *1 lemon zest and slices*
- *3 garlic cloves, chopped*
- *¼ cup basil leaves torn*

DIRECTIONS

1. Preheat the oven to 400°F.
2. Add the garlic, tomatoes, and lemon slices to a 9x13–inch baking dish. Drizzle with olive oil and toss well. Scoot to one side.
3. Pat the fish dry and put in the baking dish. Turn it to coat each side with oil. Spread out the tomato mixture to nestle in the fillets. Put the tomatoes over the fish and the lemons underneath. Season with salt, pepper, and chili flakes to taste.
4. Bake for 10 minutes. Take out and shake the pan to jostle the tomatoes. Sprinkle with lemon zest. Bake for 5 more minutes or until the fish is cooked.
5. Then, add the basil leaves and toss with the tomatoes to wilt the basil.
6. Garnish each portion with a wilted basil leaf and serve.

CEVICHE

SERVINGS: 6   PREP TIME: 25 min.   COOK TIME: 30 min.

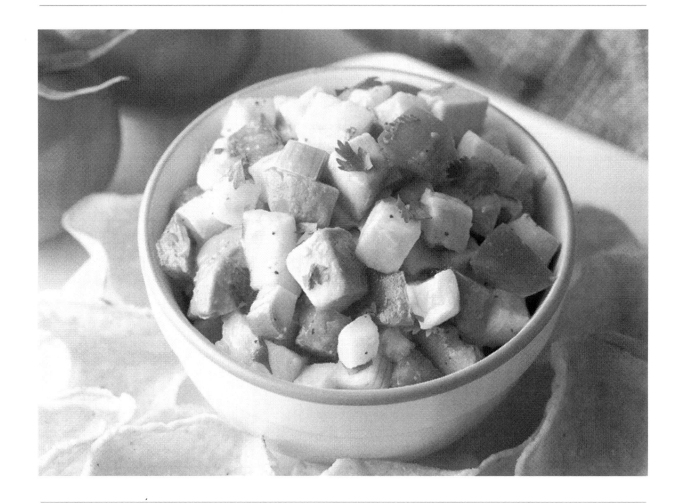

CARBS–9 g   FAT–11 g   PROTEIN–9 g   CALORIES–160

INGREDIENTS

- *1 pound fresh fish, diced into ½ inch cubes*
- *½ red onion, diced*
- *2–3 garlic cloves, minced*
- *1 jalapeño chili pepper, seeded and chopped*
- *¾ cup lime juice, squeezed*
- *1 cup cherry tomatoes, diced*
- *1 cup cucumber, diced*
- *1 Tbsp olive oil*
- *1 semi–firm avocado, diced*
- *1–1½ tsp kosher salt, more to taste*
- *¼ tsp black pepper*
- *¼–½ cup fresh cilantro chopped*

DIRECTIONS

1. Dice the onion and season with salt. Leave for 15 minutes until it releases the liquid. Rinse the onion well and squeeze dry.
2. Add the fish, onion, salt, pepper, garlic, chilies, and lime juice to a shallow bowl, and mix well. Marinate for at least 30 minutes in the fridge.
3. Before serving, gently stir in the cilantro, cucumber, avocado, tomato, and a drizzle with oil, mix carefully.

WHITE FISH WITH POTATO AND BRUSSEL SPROUT HASH

SERVINGS: 2   PREP TIME 15 min.   COOK TIME: 30 min.

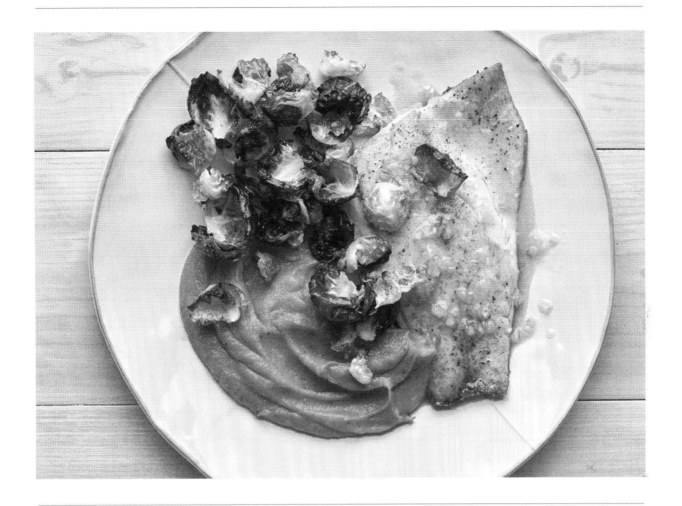

CARBS–27 g   FAT–10 g   PROTEIN–20 g   CALORIES–304

INGREDIENTS

- *2 6–ounce fish filets*
- *8 –10 ounces sweet potatoes, thinly sliced*
- *1 large shallot, sliced*
- *1 Tbsp olive oil*
- *8 ounces Brussel sprouts, thinly sliced*
- *2–4 tsp whole grain mustard*
- *2 tsp olive oil*
- *Salt and pepper to taste*

DIRECTIONS

1. Preheat the oven to 450°F.
2. Prepare a baking sheet–line it with a piece of parchment paper.
3. Toss the potatoes and shallots and with oil, salt, and pepper in a bowl. Arrange them on a lined baking sheet in one layer. Bake for 20 minutes.
4. Add the sprouts to the same bowl. Toss and sprinkle with salt and pepper to taste. Set aside.
5. Mix the mustard and oil in a small bowl. Then, season the fish fillets with salt and pepper and spoon the mustard mixture over the fish.
6. When 20 minutes have passed, add the sprouts and toss a little. Prepare a spot for the fish and place it inside. Bake for 10–12 minutes or until the fish is well–done.
7. You can puree the roasted potatoes before serving if desired
8. Garnish the fillets with the Brussel sprouts and sweet potatoes on the side and serve.

BAKED COD WITH LEMON, GARLIC AND THYME

SERVINGS: 4   PREP TIME: 15 min.   COOK TIME: 25 min.

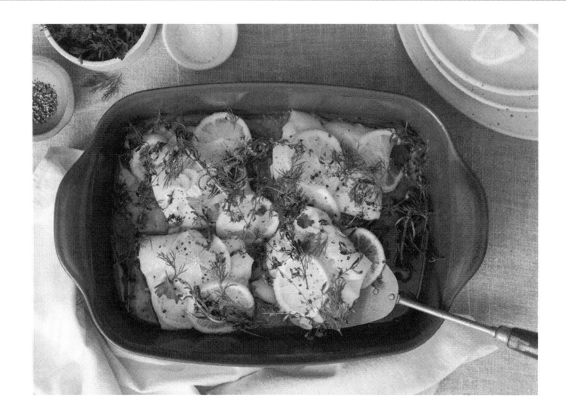

CARBS–14 g   FAT–11 g   PROTEIN–28 g   CALORIES–266

INGREDIENTS

- *2 (1–1½ lbs.) cod fillets, cut into 4 pieces*
- *1 Tbsp olive oil*
- *1 tsp kosher salt*
- *½ tsp pepper*
- *2 tsp fresh thyme*
- *1 lemon zest and slices*
- *2 Tbsp olive oil*
- *1 fennel bulb, cored and sliced*
- *1 leek, white + green parts, cut into half moons*
- *4 cloves garlic, rough chopped*
- *1 Tbsp fresh thyme*
- *½ cup chicken broth, more as needed*
- *Salt and pepper, to taste*

DIRECTIONS

1. Preheat the oven 400°F.
2. Pat the cod pieces dry. Add them to a bowl, drizzle with oil and season with salt, pepper, thyme, and zest and toss to coat. Set aside.
3. Heat 2 Tbsp of oil in a cast–iron skillet over a medium heat.
4. Add the fennel and cook for 5–7 minutes, stirring.
5. Add the leeks and garlic. Cook, stirring until tender.
6. Add the lemon zest, lemon slices, thyme, and broth. Season and simmer for 5 minutes on a medium–low heat until the liquid has reduced by half, and the fennel is tender. Add more broth if it's not and cook for a little bit longer.
7. Transfer everything into a baking dish and place the fish fillets on top. Pour all of the excess marinade over the fish. Bake for 10–15 or more until cooked through.
8. Divide among four bowls to serve. Top with lemon slice and a thyme sprig.

SHRIMP TACOS WITH MANGO CABBAGE SLAW

SERVINGS: 2   PREP TIME: 25 min.   COOK TIME: 5 min.

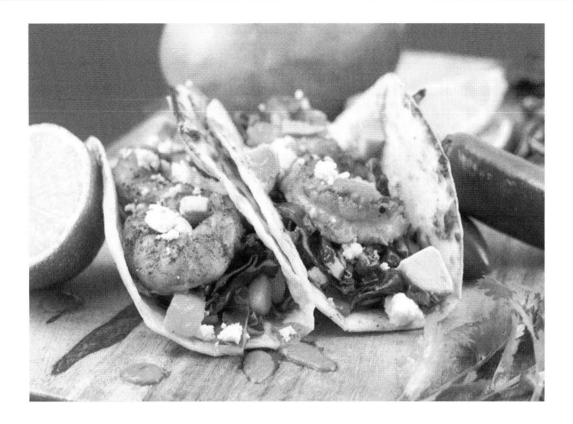

CARBS–17 g   FAT–2 g   PROTEIN–2 g   CALORIES–445

INGREDIENTS

- *1 lb. large raw shrimp, thawed, peeled and deveined*
- *1–2 tsp oil*
- *¼ tsp salt*
- *¼ tsp sugar*
- *1 tsp yellow curry powder*
- *½ tsp allspice*
- *½ tsp cinnamon*
- *½ tsp cumin*
- *½ tsp ground ginger*
- *¼ tsp cayenne or chipotle powder*
- *2 cups mango cabbage slaw*
- *6–8 (6–inch) toasted tortillas*
- *½ lime juice*

FOR THE CABBAGE SLAW:
- *3 cups thinly shredded purple cabbage*
- *1 large mango, ripe but firm, peeled and diced*
- *¼ cup red onion, finely diced*
- *2 tsp olive oil*
- *1 orange zest and juice*
- *1 lime*
- *½ tsp salt*

DIRECTIONS

1. Pat all of the shrimp dry. Drizzle with 1–2 tsp oil to lightly coat them.
2. Mix the salt, sugar, and all of the spices in a small bowl. Toss the spices with the shrimp, mixing well. Set aside.
3. To make a cabbage slaw, add the shredded cabbage and mango to a large bowl.
4. Add the onion, zest, orange juice, oil, and jalapeno. Mix to combine.
5. Put the shrimp in an oiled cast–iron skillet and grill for 45 seconds on each side over a medium–high heat. Squeeze ½ a lime over the shrimp.
6. Serve the shrimp and cabbage slaw with tortillas.

FOIL BAKED SALMON

SERVINGS: 4 PREP TIME: 10 min. COOK TIME: 25 min.

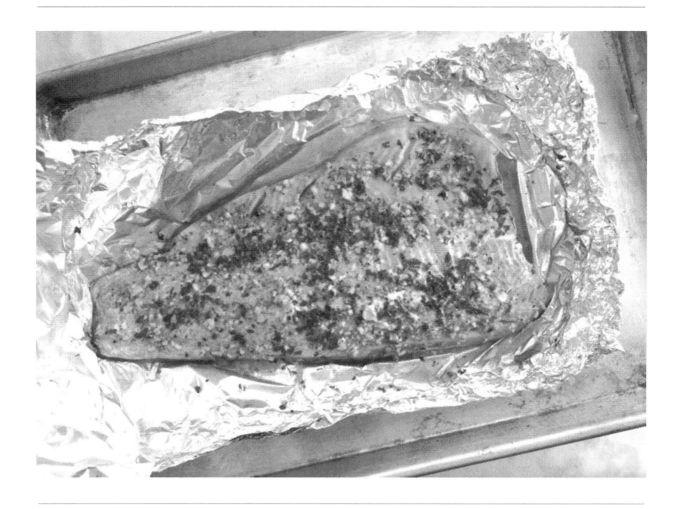

CARBS–1 g FAT–8 g PROTEIN–41 g CALORIES–256

INGREDIENTS

- *1 (3 lb.) large salmon fillet*
- *6 Tbsp butter, melted*
- *2 Tbsp honey*
- *3 cloves garlic, minced*
- *2 lemons, thinly sliced*
- *1 tsp chopped thyme leaves*
- *1 tsp dried oregano*
- *¼ cup chopped parsley*
- *Kosher salt, to taste*
- *Black pepper, to taste*

DIRECTIONS

1. Preheat the oven to 350°F.
2. Line a baking sheet using foil and use cooking spray to oil it.
3. Lay the lemon slices in one layer in the center of the foil.
4. Season the salmon with salt and pepper on both sides and transfer on top of the lemon slices.
5. Mix the butter, honey, thyme, garlic, and oregano in a small bowl.
6. Pour the butter mixture over salmon and fold up the foil around the fish.
7. Bake for 25 minutes or until the salmon is cooked through.
8. Switch to broil, and cook for 2 minutes to thicken the butter mixture.
9. Sprinkle with chopped parsley before serving.

GRILLED HALIBUT WITH MANGO SALSA

SERVINGS: 4   PREP TIME: 5 min.   COOK TIME: 20 min.

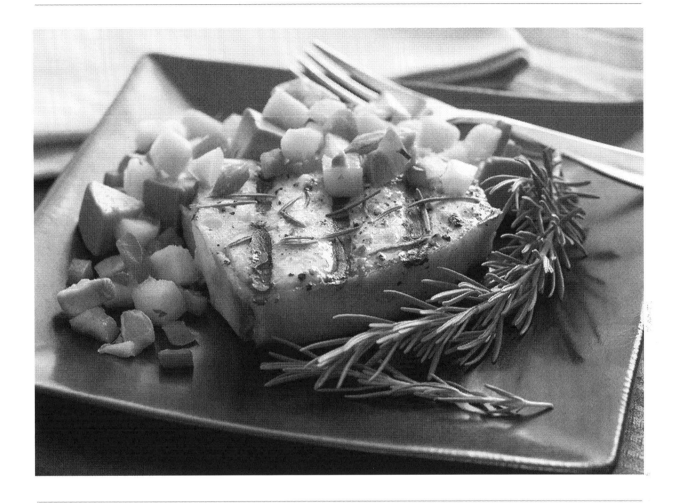

CARBS–7 g   FAT–9 g   PROTEIN–22 g   CALORIES–111

INGREDIENTS

FOR THE HALIBUT:

- *4 (4–6 oz.) halibut steaks*
- *2 Tbsp extra–virgin olive oil*
- *Kosher salt, to taste*
- *Black pepper, to taste*

FOR THE MANGO SALSA:

- *1 mango, diced*
- *1 avocado, diced*
- *1 red pepper, finely chopped*
- *½ red onion, diced*
- *1 jalapeno, minced*
- *1 Tbsp chopped cilantro*
- *1 lime juice*
- *Kosher salt, to taste*
- *Black pepper, to taste*

DIRECTIONS

1. Preheat the grill to medium–high and oil the halibut on both sides. Season with salt and pepper.
2. Grill the halibut for 5 minutes on each side or until cooked through.
3. Mix all of the ingredients for the salsa in a bowl and season with salt and pepper to taste.
4. Serve the salsa over the grilled halibut.

FISH TACOS

SERVINGS: 4   PREP TIME: 20 min.   COOK TIME: 15 min.

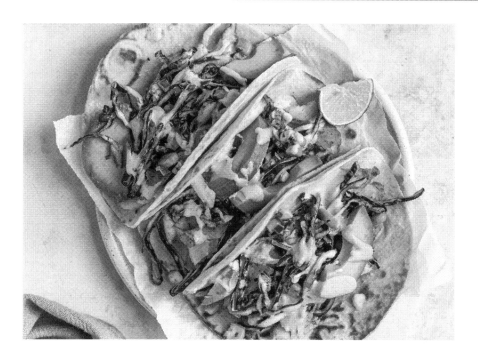

CARBS–22 g   FAT–17 g   PROTEIN–9 g   CALORIES–270

INGREDIENTS

- *3 Tbsp extra–virgin olive oil*
- *1 lime juice*
- *2 tsp chili powder*
- *1 tsp paprika*
- *½ tsp ground cumin*
- *½ tsp cayenne pepper*
- *1½ lb. cod fillets*
- *½ Tbsp vegetable oil*
- *Kosher salt, to taste*
- *Black pepper, to taste*
- *8 corn tortillas*
- *1 avocado, diced*
- *Lime wedges, for serving*
- *Sour cream, for serving*

FOR THE CORN SLAW:
- *¼ cup mayonnaise*
- *1 lime juice*
- *2 Tbsp freshly chopped cilantro*
- *1 Tbsp honey*
- *2 cups shredded purple cabbage*
- *1 cup corn kernels*
- *1 jalapeño, minced*

DIRECTIONS

1. Whisk the oil, lime juice, cumin, chili powder, paprika, and cayenne pepper in a shallow bowl.
2. Add the cod and toss to coat evenly. Leave for 15 minutes to marinate.
3. To make the slaw, whisk the mayonnaise, lime juice, cilantro, and honey in a large bowl. Add in the cabbage, corn, and jalapeno and stir well. Season with salt and pepper to taste.
4. Heat the oil over a medium–high heat in a large skillet.
5. Take the cod out of the marinade and season each filet with salt and pepper on both sides.
6. Add the fish flesh side down. Cook for 3–5 minutes per side until cooked through. Let it rest for 5 minutes, then flake with a fork.
7. Serve the fillets on grilled tortillas with avocado and corn slaw. Squeeze lime juice on top.

HONEY GARLIC SHRIMP

SERVINGS: 4   PREP TIME: 15 min.   COOK TIME: 5 min.

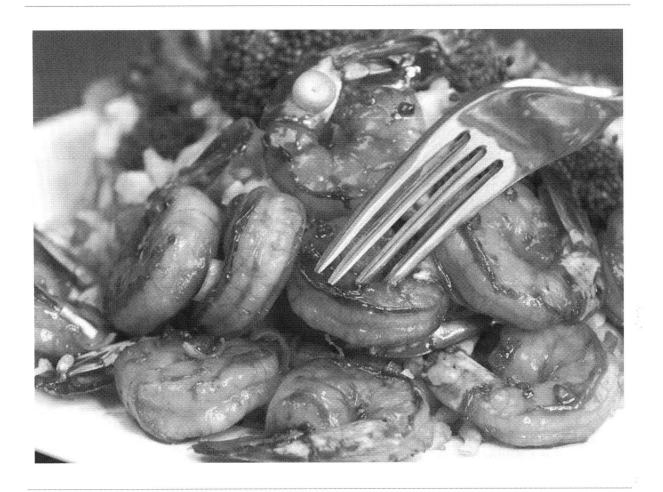

CARBS–3 g   FAT–0 g   PROTEIN–1 g   CALORIES–21

INGREDIENTS

- *⅓ cup honey*
- *¼ cup soy sauce*
- *2 tsp fresh minced garlic*
- *1 tsp minced fresh ginger*
- *1 lb. medium uncooked shrimp, peeled & deveined*
- *2 tsp olive oil*

DIRECTIONS

1. Whisk the soy sauce, honey, garlic, and ginger in a bowl.
2. Put the shrimp in a large Ziploc bag. Pour half of the marinade on top, close, and shake to coat evenly. Leave for 30 minutes to marinate in the fridge. Cover the second half of the marinade and refrigerate for later use.
3. Heat the olive oil over a medium–high heat in a skillet.
4. Discard the used marinade and add the shrimp to the skillet. Cook for 45 seconds on each side. Then, pour in the reserved marinade and cook for 1 more minute until shrimp is cooked through.
5. Serve the shrimp immediately with the cooked marinade sauce.

NORDIC NICOISE SALAD

SERVINGS: 2   PREP TIME: 15 min.   COOK TIME: 35 min.

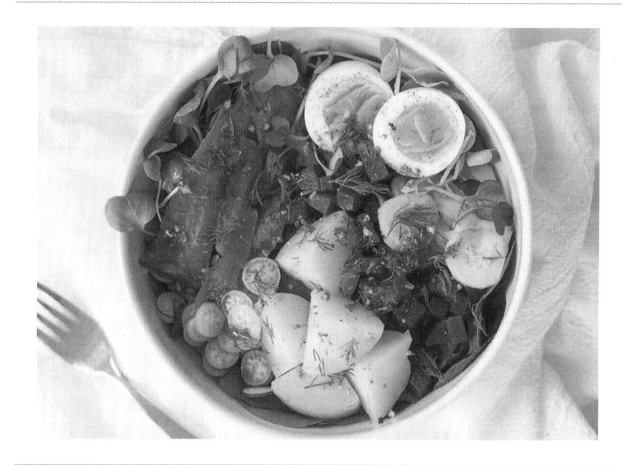

CARBS–32 g   FAT–25 g   PROTEIN–38 g   CALORIES–532

INGREDIENTS

- *8 baby potatoes or other, boiled*
- *2 eggs, boiled and halved*
- *1–2 Turkish cucumbers, shaved*
- *½ fennel bulb, shaved and slice*
- *4–6 radishes, sliced*
- *1 bunch watercress or other greens*
- *1 cup chopped jarred pickled beets*
- *6 ounces smoked salmon*
- *1 Tbsp capers (optional)*
- *Fresh dill*

FOR THE DRESSING:
- *¼ cup olive oil*
- *2 Tbsp lemon juice*
- *1 tsp whole grain mustard*
- *1 Tbsp shallot, finely chopped*
- *1 Tbsp fresh dill, chopped*
- *¼ tsp salt*
- *¼ tsp black pepper*
- *1–2 tsp fresh grated horseradish*

DIRECTIONS

1. To make the dressing, mix all of the dressing components in a small bowl with a fork.
2. Form a watercress bed on the bottom of two serving bowls. Top with cucumber, radish, fennel, salmon, eggs, onions, capers (if used), and dill.
3. Drizzle with the dressing right before serving.

TRADITIONAL CHICKEN COBB SALAD

SERVINGS: 6   PREP TIME: 20 min.   COOK TIME: 40 min.

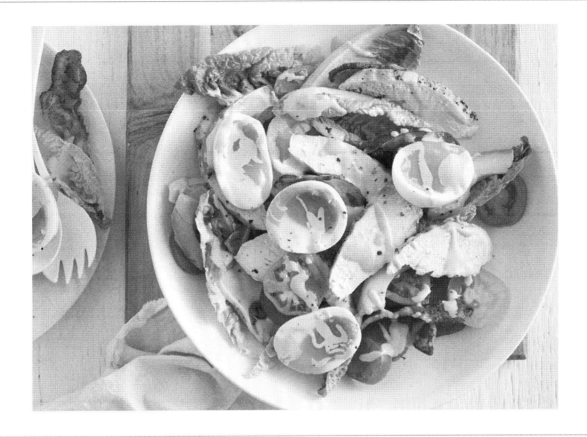

CARBS–7 g   FAT–59 g   PROTEIN–42 g   CALORIES–733

INGREDIENTS

FOR THE DRESSING:
- *1 Tbsp Dijon mustard*
- *2 Tbsp shallot, minced*
- *¼ cup lemon juice*
- *½ tsp sugar*
- *½ tsp salt*
- *¼ tsp black pepper*
- *⅓ cup olive oil*

FOR THE SALAD:
- *1 lb. boneless, skinless chicken breasts*
- *4 hard–boiled eggs*
- *½ lb. bacon, cooked*
- *1 head green leaf lettuce, torn*
- *6 tomatoes, sliced*
- *1 avocado, thinly sliced*

DIRECTIONS

1. To make the dressing, whisk the mustard, lemon juice, sugar, shallots, salt, and pepper. Slowly whisk in the olive oil until it's completely emulsified. Set aside.
2. Grease the chicken breasts with oil. Season to taste on both sides.
3. Heat an oiled skillet over a medium–high heat.
4. Add the meat and cook for 3–4 minutes per side until seared. Cover and cook for 7–10 minutes until it's cooked through. Transfer to a plate and let it rest covered with foil for 10 minutes before slicing.
5. Cut the eggs into quarters. Cut the bacon into 1–inch pieces.
6. Lay the lettuce leaves on a large plate. Top with the sliced chicken, bacon, eggs, tomatoes, and avocado.
7. Drizzle with the dressing or serve it on the side.

CHICKEN CAESAR SALAD

SERVINGS: 4   PREP TIME: 10 min.   COOK TIME: 20 min.

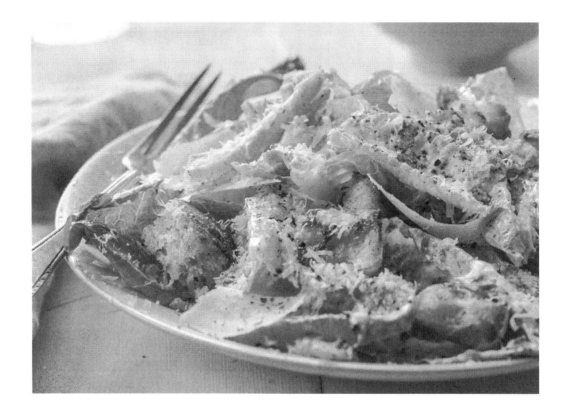

CARBS–5 g   FAT–18 g   PROTEIN–18 g   CALORIES–307

INGREDIENTS

- *4 thick slices crusty white bread*
- *3 Tbsp olive oil, divided*
- *2 skinless, boneless chicken breasts*
- *1 large romaine lettuce, leaves separated, torn*

FOR THE DRESSING:

- *1 garlic clove, minced*
- *2 anchovies from a tin, mashed*
- *⅓ cup grated Parmesan*
- *5 Tbsp mayonnaise*
- *1 Tbsp white wine vinegar*

DIRECTIONS

1. Preheat the oven to 390°F.
2. Cut the bread into cubes and arrange on a large baking sheet. Sprinkle with 2 Tbsp olive oil.
3. Rub the oil into the bread and season with sea salt if desired. Bake for 8–10 minutes, turning a few times during cooking to brown them evenly.
4. Rub the breasts with 1 Tbsp olive oil and season.
5. Heat a pan over a medium heat until it's hot. Add the chicken to the pan and cook for 4 mins.
6. Flip the chicken, and cook for 4 more minutes. Check if it's cooked and no longer pink in the thickest part.
7. Mix the cheese, garlic, anchovies, mayonnaise, and vinegar in a bowl until it's as thick as yogurt. If not, adjust with 1 Tbsp water at a time. Season with salt and pepper to taste.
8. Add the torn lettuce leaves to the bowl and toss with enough dressing. Then, arrange the leaves on a platter.
9. Top with the rest of the ingredients and serve with the rest of the dressing on the side.

CAPRESE SALAD

SERVINGS: 4   PREP TIME: 10 min.   COOK TIME: 10 min.

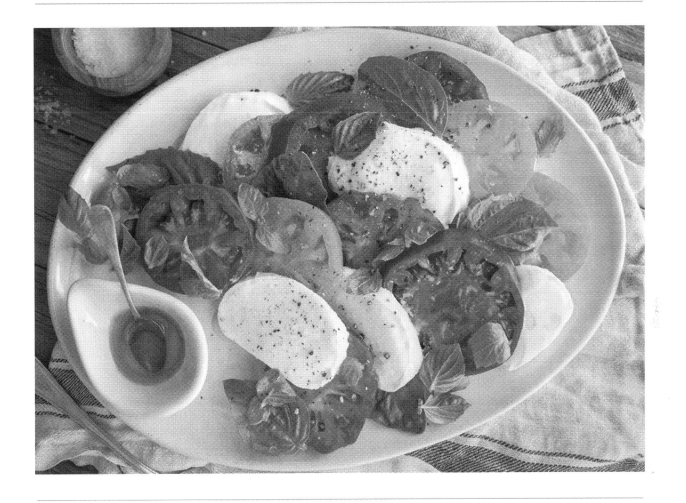

CARBS–9 g   FAT–18 g   PROTEIN–14 g   CALORIES–250

INGREDIENTS

- *3–4 medium tomatoes, sliced*
- *1 (8–ounce) ball fresh mozzarella, sliced*
- *½ cup fresh basil leaves*
- *2 Tbsp extra–virgin olive oil, for drizzling*
- *Salt and black pepper, to taste*

DIRECTIONS

1. Arrange the mozzarella, tomatoes, and basil on a platter.
2. Drizzle with oil and sprinkle with sea salt and black pepper to taste before serving.

AUTUMN APPLE SALAD WITH A MAPLE VINAIGRETTE

SERVINGS: 1   PREP TIME: 5 min.   COOK TIME: 2 h.

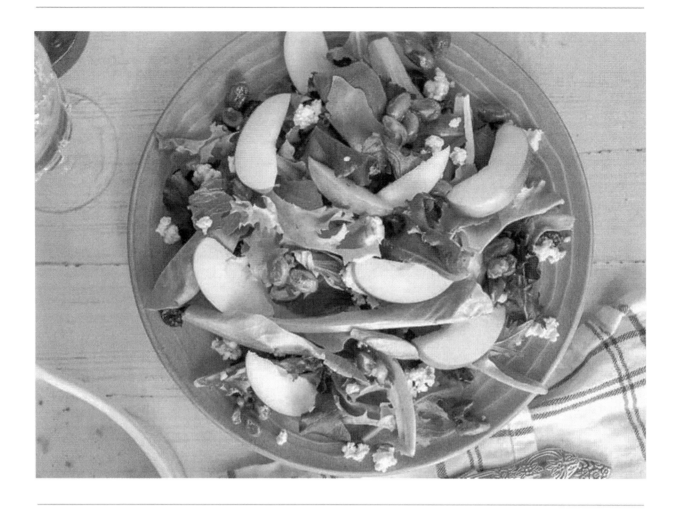

CARBS–26 g   FAT–8 g   PROTEIN–4 g   CALORIES–284

INGREDIENTS

- *2 cups optional leafy greens*
- *¼ cup dried cranberries*
- *¼ cup nuts of choice*
- *2 Tbsp feta cheese, crumbled*
- *½ granny smith apple, sliced*
- *½ Fuji apple, sliced*
- *2 slices bacon, cooked and chopped*

FOR THE DRESSING:
- *2 Tbsp extra virgin olive oil*
- *1 Tbsp apple cider vinegar*
- *1 Tbsp maple syrup*
- *1½ tsp Dijon mustard*
- *Salt and black pepper to taste*

DIRECTIONS

1. Add the leafy greens to a large bowl.
2. Top with the nuts, cheese, apples, and bacon.
3. Add all of the components for the dressing to a mason jar. Close and shake to mix.
4. Pour the dressing over the salad and serve.

CRUNCHY TURKEY SALAD

SERVINGS: 6   PREP TIME: 10 min.   COOK TIME: 10 min.

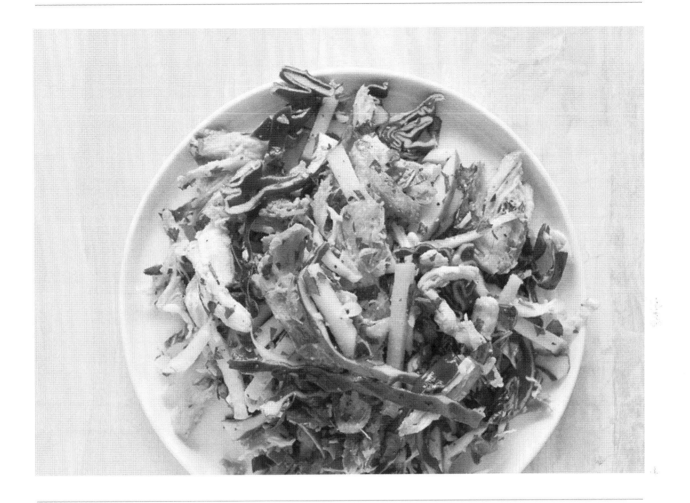

CARBS–19 g   FAT–11 g   PROTEIN–14 g   CALORIES–227

INGREDIENTS

- *1 pound turkey breast, shredded*
- *½ head red cabbage, shredded*
- *½ head white cabbage, shredded*
- *1 bell pepper, de–seeded and sliced*
- *1 large carrot cut into matchsticks*
- *3 green onions, finely sliced*
- *4 Tbsp chopped cilantro*
- *3 Tbsp toasted sesame seeds*
- *3 Tbsp toasted nuts optional*

FOR THE DRESSING:
- *¼ cup tahini*
- *¼ cup water, more if needed*
- *¼ cup lemon juice*
- *1 garlic clove minced*
- *Sweetener to taste*
- *Salt to taste*
- *Black pepper to taste*

DIRECTIONS

1. Add all of the salad components to a large bowl and mix well to combine.
2. To make the dressing, add all of the ingredients for it in a blender and blend for 30 seconds–1 minute until creamy.
3. Add half of the dressing into the salad bowl and toss well to coat evenly. Adjust the salt and pepper to taste, if needed.

CHINESE CHICKEN SALAD

SERVINGS: 6   PREP TIME: 10 min.   COOK TIME: 5 min.

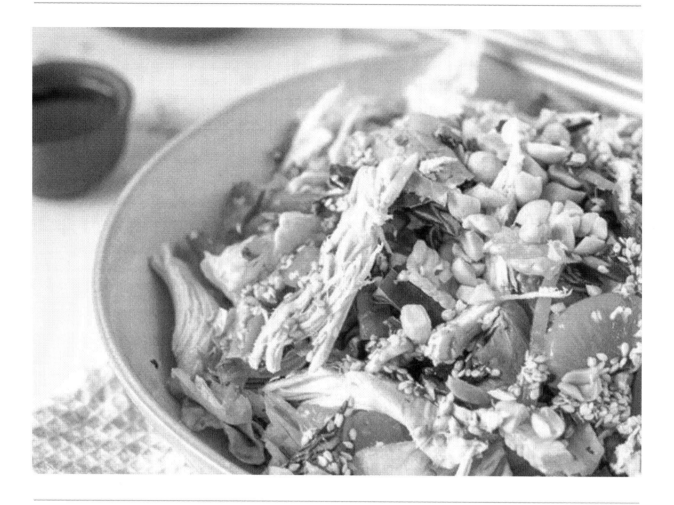

CARBS–17 g   FAT–13 g   PROTEIN–27 g   CALORIES–307

INGREDIENTS

FOR THE DRESSING:
- 2 Tbsp canola oil
- ⅓ cup rice vinegar
- ¼ cup hoisin sauce
- 1½ Tbsp soy sauce
- 1 Tbsp fresh ginger, grated
- ½ tsp toasted sesame oil

FOR THE SALAD:
- 4 cups cooked chicken, shredded
- 2 cups red cabbage, cored and finely shredded
- 1 pound Napa cabbage, cored and shredded
- 1 cup carrots, shredded
- 1 bunch scallions, thinly sliced
- ¼ cup fresh cilantro, minced
- 1 cup chow mein noodles (optional)
- 2 Tbsp sesame seeds for garnish

DIRECTIONS

1. To make the dressing, whisk the vinegar, oil, soy sauce, hoisin sauce, ginger, and sesame oil in a small bowl. Leave it for 15 minutes.
2. Also, you can store the dressing in the fridge for up to 3–4 days.
3. Mix the chicken, carrots, green and red cabbage, scallions, and cilantro in a bowl.
4. Drizzle with the dressing and toss to combine. Sprinkle with sesame seeds and noodles, if using.

GREEK SALAD

SERVINGS: 4   PREP TIME: 15 min.   COOK TIME: 15 min.

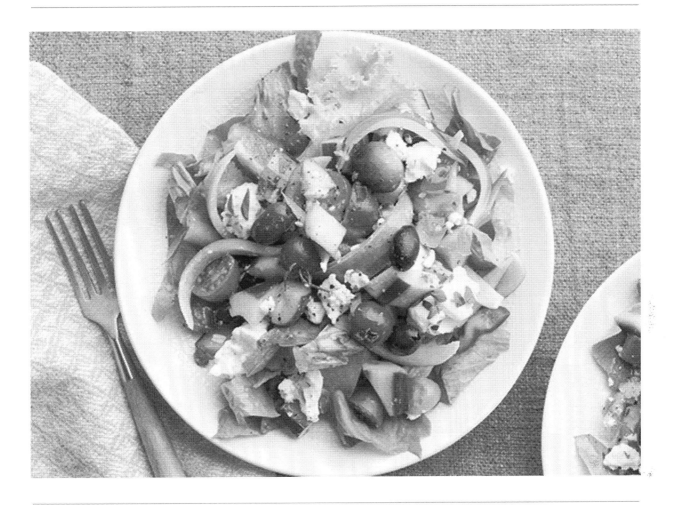

CARBS–10 g   FAT–9 g   PROTEIN–9 g   CALORIES–142

INGREDIENTS

FOR THE DRESSING:
- ¼ cup extra–virgin olive oil
- 3 Tbsp red wine vinegar
- 1 garlic clove, minced
- ½ tsp dried oregano
- ¼ tsp Dijon mustard
- ¼ tsp sea salt
- Black pepper, to taste

FOR THE SALAD:
- 1 English cucumber, quartered and sliced
- 2 cups cherry tomatoes, sliced
- ⅓ cup reddish, sliced
- 5 ounces feta cheese, cut into cubes
- ⅓ cup red onion, thinly sliced
- ⅓ cup pitted Kalamata olives
- ⅓ cup fresh mint leaves

DIRECTIONS

1. To make the dressing, whisk the olive oil, garlic, oregano, vinegar, mustard, salt, and pepper in a small bowl.
2. Mix the cucumber, green pepper, tomatoes, cheese, red onions, and olives in a large bowl. Drizzle the salad with dressing and gently toss.
3. Arrange the salad on a serving platter and mint leaves if desired. Season to taste and serve.

GRILLED POTATO SALAD WITH GRILLED SCALLION VINAIGRETTE

SERVINGS: 4   PREP TIME: 15 min.   COOK TIME: 30 min.

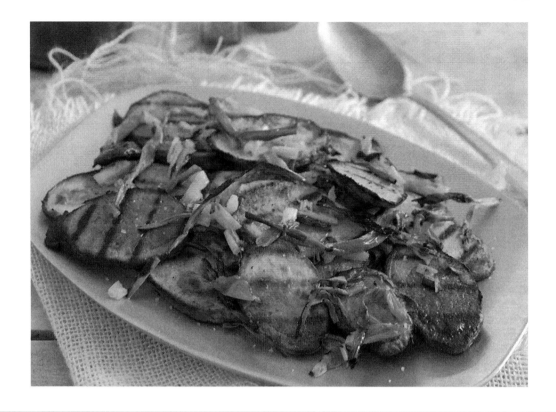

CARBS–23 g   FAT–16 g   PROTEIN–3 g   CALORIES–240

INGREDIENTS

- *2 pounds tiny potatoes or fingerling potatoes*
- *Extra–virgin olive oil, for drizzling*
- *¼ cup fresh mint leaves*
- *⅓ cup pickled onions, optional*
- *2 scallions, finely chopped*
- *Sea salt, to taste*

FOR THE DRESSING:
- *1 bunch scallions*
- *2½ Tbsp extra–virgin olive oil*
- *1 Tbsp champagne vinegar*
- *1 Tbsp white miso*
- *½ Tbsp Dijon mustard*
- *2 Tbsp water*
- *1 tsp hot sauce of your choice*
- *Sea salt, to taste*

DIRECTIONS

1. Fill a medium pot with water (room temperature). Add salt to the water and then add the potatoes. Bring to a boil, then simmer on low. Cook for 15 minutes until fork–tender. You will finish them later on the grill. Drain, and cool enough to handle. Slice the potatoes lengthwise.
2. Preheat a grill to medium heat.
3. Meanwhile, toss the scallions with ½ Tbsp oil and a pinch of salt to make a dressing. Grill them for 1 minute and then flip. Chop and put into a food processor. Add the miso, vinegar, mustard, hot sauce, and 3 Tbsp water. Pulse to combine well. Add cilantro and 2 Tbsp oil, and pulse one more time.
4. Toss the potatoes with oil, salt, and pepper. Grill for 2–4 minutes to form marks. Flip, and cook for 3 minutes or so, until they are well charred and tender. The time depends on the size of the potatoes.
5. Assemble the salad with potatoes, dressing, mint, and chopped scallions.
6. Serve warm or at room temperature.

CUCUMBER LETTUCE SALAD

SERVINGS: 4   PREP TIME: 15 min.   COOK TIME: 15 min.

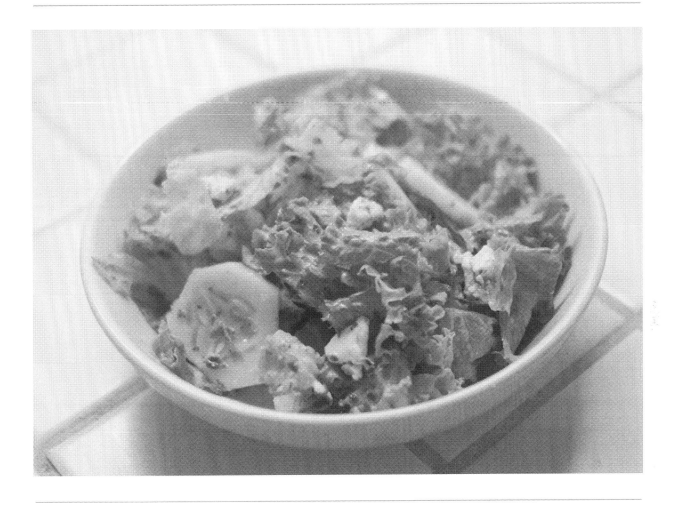

CARBS–1 g   FAT–1 g   PROTEIN–2 g   CALORIES–38

INGREDIENTS

FOR THE SALAD:
- 5 ounces lettuce salad
- 1 English cucumber, sliced
- ½ medium red onion, sliced (optional)

FOR THE DRESSING:
- 3 Tbsp olive oil
- 1 Tbsp freshly–squeezed lemon juice
- 1 tsp Dijon mustard
- 1 small clove garlic, finely minced
- ½ tsp fine sea salt
- ¼ tsp freshly–cracked black pepper

DIRECTIONS

1. To make the dressing, whisk all of the ingredients in a bowl until well combined.
2. Combine all of the salad components in a large salad bowl.
3. Drizzle with the dressing and toss until evenly combined.
4. Serve immediately.

SPINACH RICE

SERVINGS: 3   PREP TIME: 10 min.   COOK TIME: 20 min.

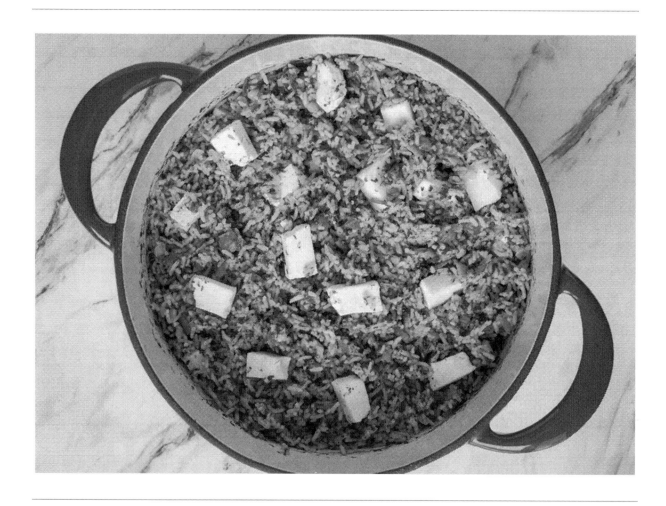

CARBS–18 g   FAT–14 g   PROTEIN–7 g   CALORIES–350

INGREDIENTS

- *1 cup white rice, rinsed and drained*
- *2–3 cups fresh baby spinach*
- *2 tomatoes, diced*
- *1 medium onion, diced*
- *2–3 cloves garlic, minced*
- *2 cups vegetable stock low sodium or water*
- *1½ tsp curry powder*
- *1 tsp cooking oil*
- *Tofu, for topping (optional)*
- *Salt and pepper, to taste*

DIRECTIONS

1. Heat the oil in a large skillet over a medium heat.
2. Add in the garlic. Cook for 30 seconds until fragrant.
3. Add the onion and cook for 3–4 minutes.
4. Add in the tomatoes and cook for 3–4 more minutes.
5. Add the spinach and rice, and cook for 2–3 minutes. Add the stock and let it boil.
6. Season with curry powder, salt, and pepper to taste.
7. Simmer covered for 18–20 minutes or until the rice is tender on low heat.
8. Turn off, top with tofu, and serve warm.

SPICY CORN SOUP

SERVINGS: 2   PREP TIME: 10 min.   COOK TIME: 15 min.

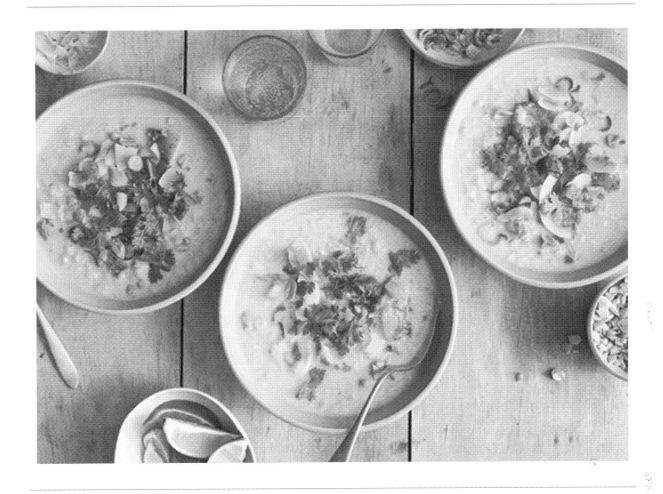

CARBS—47 g   FAT—17 g   PROTEIN—20 g   CALORIES—414

INGREDIENTS

- *1 cup milk*
- *1 cup vegetable broth*
- *1 large knob butter*
- *½ medium onion, diced*
- *1 Tbsp all–purpose flour*
- *1 can sweet corn, drained and rinsed*
- *½ red bell pepper*
- *1 chili pepper, finely chopped*
- *1 tsp cumin*
- *2 tsp curry powder*
- *½ cup cheddar cheese*
- *2 shallots (or spring onions)*
- *½ cup chopped parsley*
- *More corn, for serving*

DIRECTIONS

1. Heat the vegetable broth and milk in a pot over low heat. DO NOT boil or the fat will separate itself from the milk.
2. Heat another pot and melt the butter.
3. Add the onions and let it simmer for 3–4 minutes, then add the flour. Mix well.
4. Add the pepper, chili, and corn. Give it a stir.
5. Pour in the broth and milk mix to the pot with the vegetables. Stir in the cumin and curry powder.
6. Mix well to combine and simmer for 5 minutes on a low heat.
7. Stir in the cheddar cheese and let it melt.
8. Top with parsley and more corn.
9. You can add potatoes to the soup, but it's optional.

SWEET POTATOES WITH MISO

SERVINGS: 4–6 PREP TIME: 15 min. COOK TIME: 40 min.

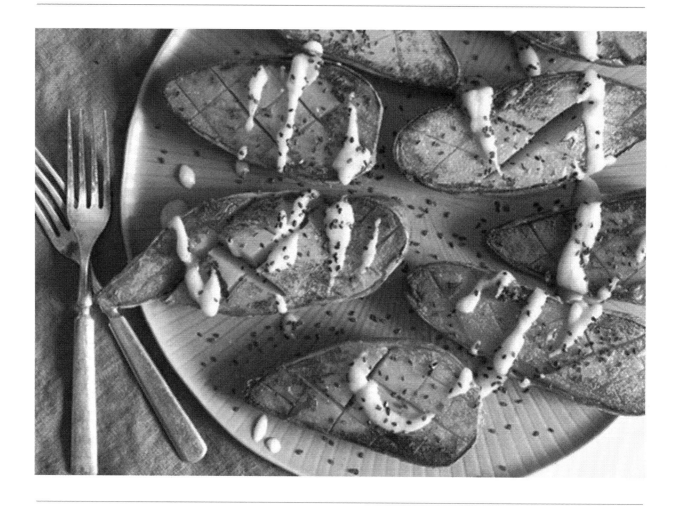

CARBS–44 g FAT–10 g PROTEIN–3 g CALORIES–271

INGREDIENTS

- *2–3 yams or small sweet potatoes, halved lengthwise*
- *Olive oil for brushing*
- *¼ cup butter or ghee*
- *1 large shallot, very finely diced*
- *2 tsp ginger, minced*
- *1 Tbsp miso*
- *Salt, to taste*
- *1 Tbsp toasted sesame seeds (optional)*

DIRECTIONS

1. Preheat the oven to 425°F.
2. Arrange the sweet potatoes on a lined sheet pan. Brush the skin side with olive oil.
3. Bake for 30–40 minutes or more until fork tender. Then, flip the potatoes over and broil for 4–5 minutes for caramelization.
4. Heat the butter in a pan over a medium–low heat.
5. Add the shallots and cook for 5–6 minutes, stirring until golden.
6. Add the ginger, cook for 2–3 more minutes.
7. Add the miso and using a fork, mash, and it into mixture, breaking it up. Cook for 2 minutes, then turn off the heat.
8. Once the potatoes are caramelized, place them on a platter and make few crisscross cuts. Spoon the miso butter over sweet potato halves.
9. Sprinkle with salt to taste and sesame seeds if desired. Serve.

VEGETARIAN FRIED RICE

SERVINGS: 2   PREP TIME: 5 min.   COOK TIME: 10 min.

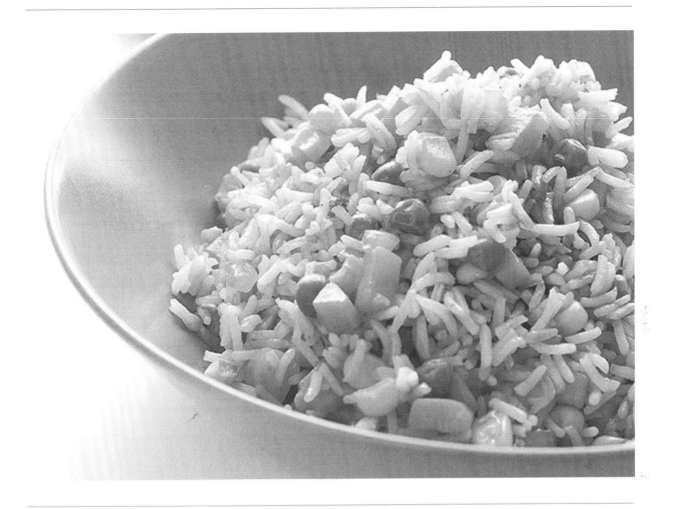

CARBS–82 g   FAT–25 g   PROTEIN–17 g   CALORIES–619

INGREDIENTS

FOR THE SAUCE:
- 2 Tbsp dark soy sauce
- 2 tsp vinegar
- 2 tsp olive oil
- 1 tsp maple syrup

FOR THE FRIED RICE:
- 2 eggs, beaten
- Salt, to taste
- 2 Tbsp sesame oil
- 3 cups cooked rice
- 1 onion, chopped
- 2 cup vegetables of choice, chopped

DIRECTIONS

1. Mix the ingredients for the sauce in a bowl.
2. Heat 1 Tbsp of sesame oil over a high heat in a pan.
3. Pour in the beaten egg and cook for 1 minute, scrambling it. While scrambling, season with salt and vinegar. Transfer to a plate and set aside.
4. Heat 1 Tbsp of oil in the pan over a high heat.
5. Add the onion and fry for 30 seconds.
6. Then, stir in the vegetables. Continue cooking for 3–5 minutes.
7. Reduce the heat, add the rice, sauce, and eggs. Stir well to combine.
8. Divide between two bowls and serve while hot.

VEGAN JAMBALAYA

SERVINGS: 6   PREP TIME: 25 minutes.   COOK TIME: 30 min.

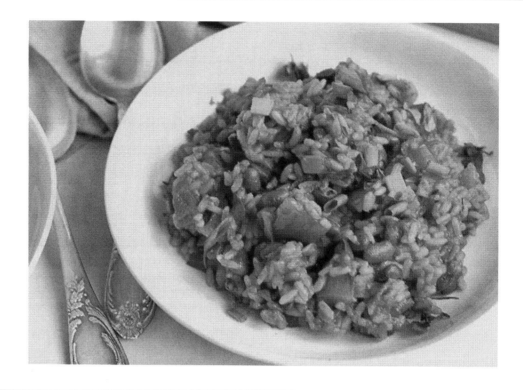

CARBS–70 g   FAT–1 g   PROTEIN–11 g   CALORIES–331

INGREDIENTS

- *1 onion, diced*
- *4 garlic cloves, minced*
- *1 celery stalk, diced*
- *½ red pepper, diced*
- *½ green pepper, diced*
- *1 can crushed tomatoes*
- *4 cups vegetable stock*
- *2 cups uncooked long grain white rice*
- *1½ cup cooked kidney beans*
- *1 tsp dried oregano*
- *1 tsp dried basil*
- *1 tsp dried thyme*
- *1 tsp sweet paprika*
- *2 tsp smoky paprika*
- *½ tsp cayenne pepper*
- *2 bay leaves*
- *2 Tbsp Tabasco sauce or to taste*
- *2 Tbsp soy sauce*
- *pepper to taste*
- *1 tsp salt adjust to taste*
- *1 handful green onion, chopped*

DIRECTIONS

1. Heat 1 Tbsp of oil over a medium–high heat in a large pan.
2. Add the onion and garlic and cook for 3–4 minutes until soft.
3. Add the celery and peppers and cook until just starting to soften.
4. Push the vegetables to one side of the pan. Cook for 3–5 more minutes until browned.
5. Add the stock, tomatoes, spices, herbs, sauces, rice, and beans. Let it boil and turn to low. Cover with a lid and simmer for 15–20 minutes.
6. When the rice is tender, adjust with salt if needed.
7. Serve with green onions on top and Tabasco sauce.

VEGETABLES TACOS

SERVINGS: 3–6   PREP TIME: 15 min.   COOK TIME: 20 min.

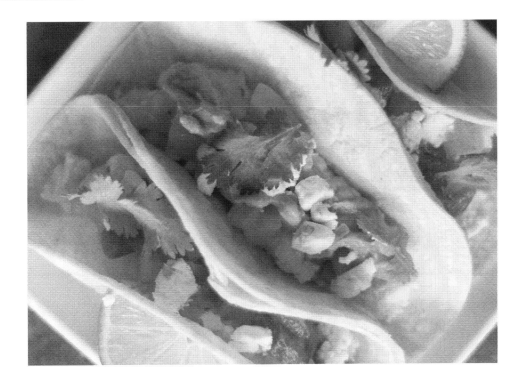

CARBS–10 g   FAT–8 g   PROTEIN–2 g   CALORIES–240

INGREDIENTS

FOR THE FILLING:

- *2 tsp olive oil*
- *1 small white or yellow onion, diced*
- *3 garlic cloves, minced*
- *1 small zucchini, sliced into 2–inch strips*
- *1 small yellow squash, sliced into 2–inch strips*
- *1 red pepper, chopped*
- *½ lime juice*
- *1 pinch red pepper flakes*
- *6 eggs, scrambled*
- *Hot sauce, to taste*
- *Salt and black pepper, to taste*
- *1 tomato, chopped*
- *6 small tortillas*

OPTIONAL GARNISHES:

- *1 jalapeño, seeded and minced*
- *Feta, crumbled*
- *Fresh cilantro, chopped*
- *Hot sauce, to taste*

DIRECTIONS

1. Heat 2 tsp of olive oil over a medium heat in a large skillet.
2. Add the onions and salt. Cook for 3–5 minutes, stirring occasionally.
3. Add the garlic and flakes. Cook for 30 seconds.
4. Add the zucchini, squash, and pepper. Cook for 7 more minutes, stirring often until the squash is cooked through and not mushy. Remove from the heat and squeeze the lime over the vegetables. Season with salt and stir well to combine. Set aside.
5. Scramble the eggs in a bowl with hot sauce, black pepper, and salt.
6. Scramble in the pan over a medium–low heat until lightly set. Fold in the tomatoes and remove the egg mixture to a bowl.
7. Warm each tortilla in a pan over a medium heat, flipping it. Transfer to a plate. Top each one with eggs, vegetables, jalapeño, feta, and cilantro.
8. Finish with your favorite hot sauce.

SPAGHETTI AGLIO E OLIO

SERVINGS: 2   PREP TIME: 5 min.   COOK TIME: 15 min.

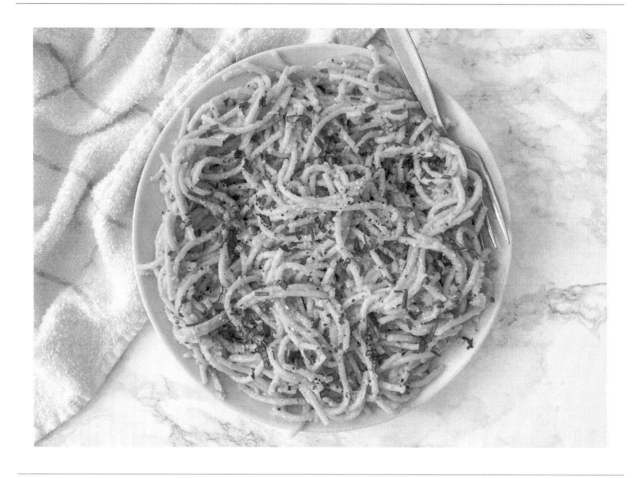

CARBS–38 g   FAT–51 g   PROTEIN–7 g   CALORIES–650

INGREDIENTS

- *2 oz dried spaghetti*
- *3 cloves garlic, minced*
- *3 Tbsp olive oil*
- *1 pinch red pepper flakes (optional)*
- *Salt and black pepper, to taste*
- *2 Tbsp fresh Italian parsley, chopped*
- *¼ cup vegan parmesan*

DIRECTIONS

1. Bring the water to a boil in a pot and salt it.
2. Add the spaghetti, and cook for 9–12 minutes, stirring until al dente.
3. Reserve ½ cup of cooking water, then drain the pasta and transfer it to a bowl.
4. Heat the oil and garlic in a pan over a medium–low heat. Cook for 10 minutes, stirring until the garlic is golden brown. Set aside.
5. Add the cooked pasta, 1 Tbsp reserved water, and chili flakes to the pan. Toss it in oil.
6. Sprinkle the parsley, half of the cheese, and mix well until cheese has melted.
7. Taste and adjust with salt and pepper.
8. Sprinkle with more parsley and vegan cheese, and serve.

MEDITERRANEAN CHICKPEA SALAD

SERVINGS: 4   PREP TIME: 15 min.   COOK TIME: 15 min.

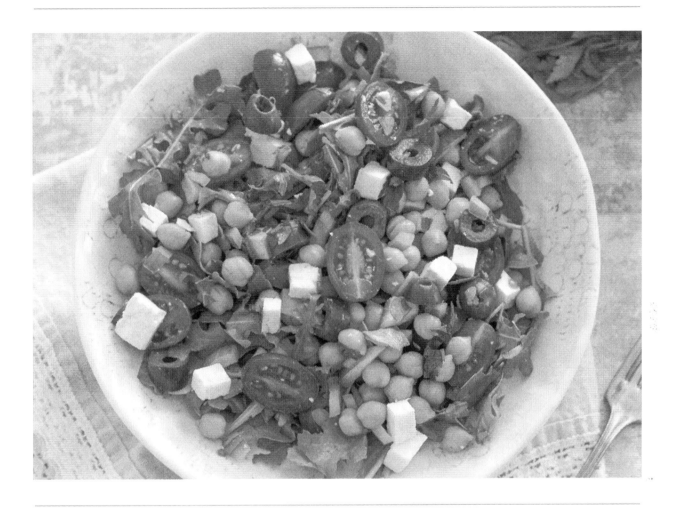

CARBS–40 g   FAT–14 g   PROTEIN–14 g   CALORIES–344

INGREDIENTS

FOR THE PESTO:
- 3 cups spinach
- 5 large basil leaves
- 1 large lemon juice
- 2 Tbsp olive oil
- 2 Tbsp Roasted Salted Blue Diamond Almonds
- 1 Tbsp grated parmesan cheese
- 3 garlic cloves, peeled
- 1–2 Tbsp water, to thin pesto
- Salt and pepper, to taste

FOR THE SALAD:
- 2 cans chickpeas, rinsed and drained
- 2 cups mixed greens of choice (lettuce, arugula)
- 1 cup grape tomatoes, halved
- ¼ cup red onion, diced
- ¼ cup pitted Kalamata olives
- ¼ cup feta, crumbled

DIRECTIONS

1. Add the spinach, almonds, basil, olive oil, lemon juice, cheese, garlic, and 1 Tbsp water in a high–powered blender. Process for 1 minute until it's smooth. Adjust the thickness with another Tbsp of water if needed. Season with salt and pepper to taste.
2. To make the salad, add the tomatoes, chickpeas, onion, and olives to a large bowl. Add in the pesto and toss to coat evenly.
3. Sprinkle crumbled feta on top and serve.

SESAME CHICKPEA STIR-FRY

SERVINGS: 4   PREP TIME: 15 min.   COOK TIME: 25 min.

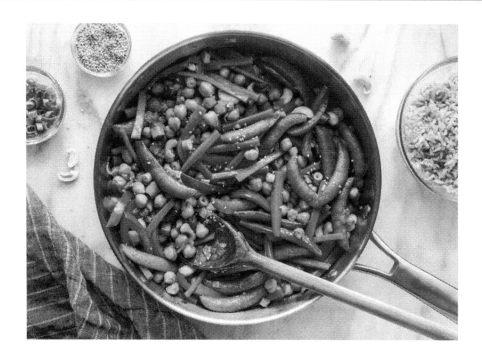

CARBS–41 g   FAT–6 g   PROTEIN–8 g   CALORIES–248

INGREDIENTS

FOR THE SAUCE:
- *¾ cup squeezed orange juice*
- *1 Tbsp honey*
- *2 Tbsp gluten free soy sauce*
- *1 tsp freshly grated ginger*
- *1 Tbsp cornstarch*
- *1 orange zest*

FOR THE STIR-FRY:
- *1 can chickpeas, rinsed and drained*
- *1½ Tbsp toasted sesame oil*
- *½ red onion, coarsely chopped*
- *3 garlic cloves, minced*
- *1 red bell pepper, sliced into strips*
- *4 oz fresh snow peas*
- *Green onion, for garnish*
- *Toasted sesame seeds, for garnish*

DIRECTIONS

1. To make the sauce, add the honey, orange juice and zest, ginger, soy sauce, cornstarch to a large bowl. Whisk to dissolve the cornstarch. Set aside.
2. Heat 1 Tbsp sesame oil over medium–high in a large skillet.
3. Add the chickpeas and cook for 5 minutes, stirring until slightly golden brown. Put into a large bowl and set aside.
4. Heat ½ Tbsp sesame oil in the same pan over a medium heat.
5. Add the onion and fry until translucent for 3–4 minutes.
6. Add the garlic and pepper. Cook for 3 minutes until slightly softened.
7. Add the snow peas and cook for 3–4 minutes.
8. Pour the sauce into the pan and stir until sauce starts to get thicker.
9. Add the chickpeas and stir again. Reduce to a medium–low heat and simmer for 3–4 minutes and thicken some more.
10. Garnish with toasted sesame seeds and green onion.

BUTTERNUT SQUASH PATTIES WITH CRANBERRY ORANGE SAUCE

SERVINGS: 4 PREP TIME: 15 min. COOK TIME: 25 min.

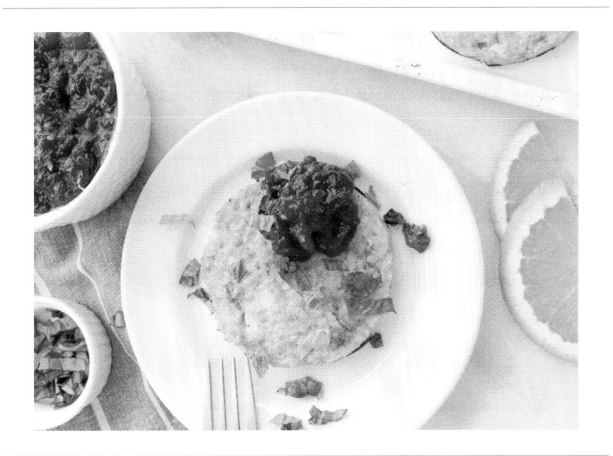

CARBS–41 g FAT–4 g PROTEIN–7 g CALORIES–231

INGREDIENTS

- 1 cup mashed and cooked butternut squash
- 1 cup cooked quinoa
- ½ small yellow onion, diced
- 2 cloves garlic, minced
- 1 egg
- ¼ tsp cumin
- ¼ cup grated parmesan cheese
- 2 Tbsp chopped basil
- Salt and pepper, to taste

FOR THE SAUCE:
- ½ pound fresh cranberries, rinsed
- ½ cup freshly squeezed orange juice
- 3 Tbsp pure maple syrup
- Non-stick cooking spray

DIRECTIONS

1. Mix the cranberries, orange juice, and maple syrup in a saucepan. Heat on high until it starts to boil, then reduce the heat to medium–low, cover and cook for 10–15 minutes until it becomes thick. Remove from the heat and let it cool.
2. Mix the quinoa, squash, egg, garlic, onion, cumin, parmesan, basil, salt and pepper in a large bowl.
3. Form 4 patties and put in the fridge for 10 minutes to help them keep their shape.
4. Heat a skillet over a medium heat, then oil it with cooking spray.
5. Add the patties to the pan and cook for 4–6 minutes until golden brown, flip and cook for 4–5 more minutes until there are crispy golden edges.
6. Serve warm with cranberry sauce over the top and sprinkled with chopped basil.

ROASTED VEGETABLES WITH OLIVE OIL AND GARLIC

SERVINGS: 8   PREP TIME: 15 min.   COOK TIME: 45 min.

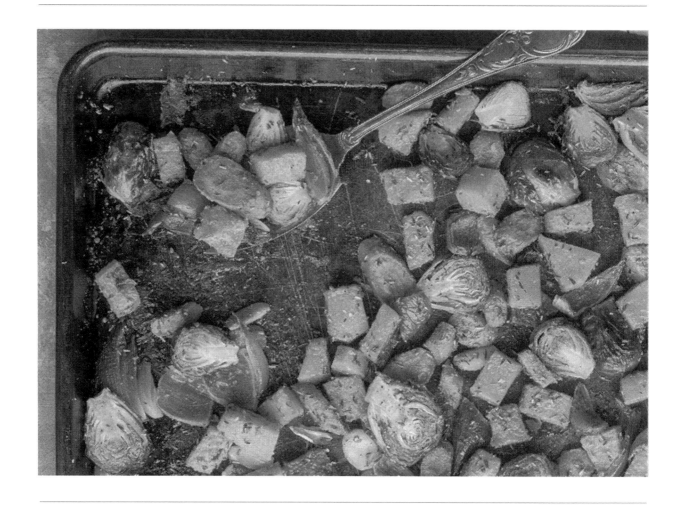

CARBS–27 g   FAT–4 g   PROTEIN–5 g   CALORIES–154

INGREDIENTS

- *1 butternut squash, peeled, seeded and cubed*
- *1 pound brussels sprouts, halved*
- *3 large carrots, peeled and sliced*
- *2 large parsnips, peeled and sliced*
- *1 large red onion, chopped*
- *12 garlic cloves, peeled*
- *2 Tbsp olive oil*
- *1 Tbsp dried oregano*
- *1 Tbsp dried rosemary*
- *¼ tsp garlic powder*
- *¼ cup Vegan Parmesan, grated*
- *½ tsp kosher salt*
- *Black pepper, to taste*

DIRECTIONS

1. Preheat the oven to 400°F.
2. Add all of the vegetables to a large bowl.
3. Whisk the olive oil, oregano, rosemary, and garlic in a small bowl. Pour over the vegetables and toss to coat. Add in the cheese, salt, pepper, and toss one more time.
4. Spread the vegetables evenly on a baking sheet. Roast for 35–45 minutes in the oven, stirring every 15–20 minutes until sprouts the sprouts have caramelized, and the squash is fork–tender.
5. Remove the vegetables from the oven, let it cool for 5 minutes and serve.

FRO-YO FRUIT BITES

SERVINGS: 12   PREP TIME: 10 min.   COOK TIME: 5 h. 10 min.

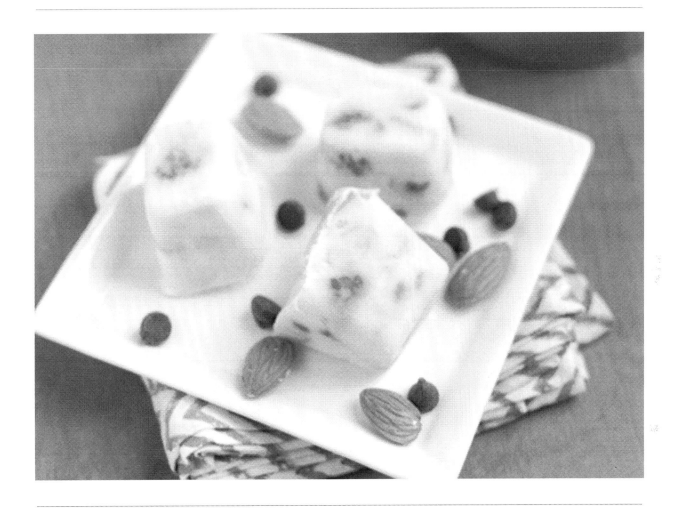

CARBS–26 g   FAT–2 g   PROTEIN–6 g   CALORIES–140

INGREDIENTS

- *1½ cups plain yogurt*
- *¼ cup whole milk*
- *2 tsp honey*
- *½ tsp pure vanilla extract*
- *2 cups fruit and berries of choice*
- *1 pinch of chocolate ships and almonds, for serving*

DIRECTIONS

1. Mix the yogurt, milk, honey, and vanilla in a bowl and whisk until smooth.
2. Arrange the fruit and berries in each mold.
3. Spoon the yogurt mixture over the fruit to fill the molds completely.
4. Freeze for about 5 hours until frozen solid.
5. Serve with chocolate chips and almonds if desired.

FROZEN STRAWBERRY CAKE

SERVINGS: 18   PREP TIME: 5 min.   COOK TIME: 25 min.

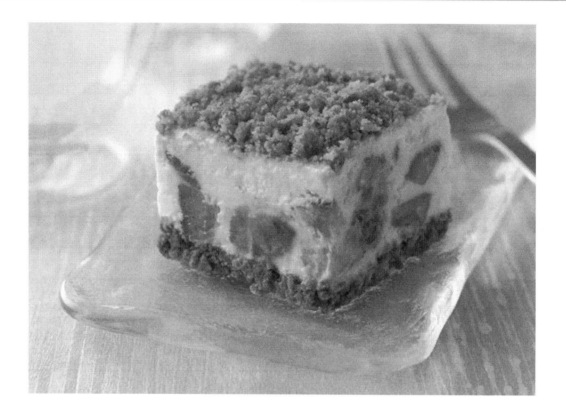

CARBS–14 g   FAT–9 g   PROTEIN–2 g   CALORIES–130

INGREDIENTS

FOR THE CRUMBS:

- 6 Tbsp ghee, melted
- 1½ cups oat flour
- ½ cup coconut sugar
- ¾ cup pecans, finely chopped

FOR THE FILLING:

- 2 egg whites
- ¾ cup granulated sweetener of choice
- 15 oz. frozen whole strawberries, partially thawed
- 2 Tbsp lemon juice

DIRECTIONS

1. Preheat the oven to 375°F.
2. Mix all of the crumb ingredients together in a large bowl.
3. Arrange the crumbs evenly on a baking sheet and bake for 15–20 minutes, stirring twice until golden brown.
4. Meanwhile, place all of the filling ingredients in the stand mixer large mixing bowl and beat for 10 minutes on high until it thickens.
5. When the crumbs are done, spread them in the bottom of a 9x13–inch pan. Reserve 1 cup for the top.
6. Pour the filling over the crumb base and smooth it.
7. Sprinkle with the reserved crumbs.
8. Freeze it for 4 hours until set.
9. Cut into portions and serve.

PEANUT BUTTER CHOCOLATE BARS

SERVINGS: 16   PREP TIME: 10 min.   COOK TIME: 20 min.

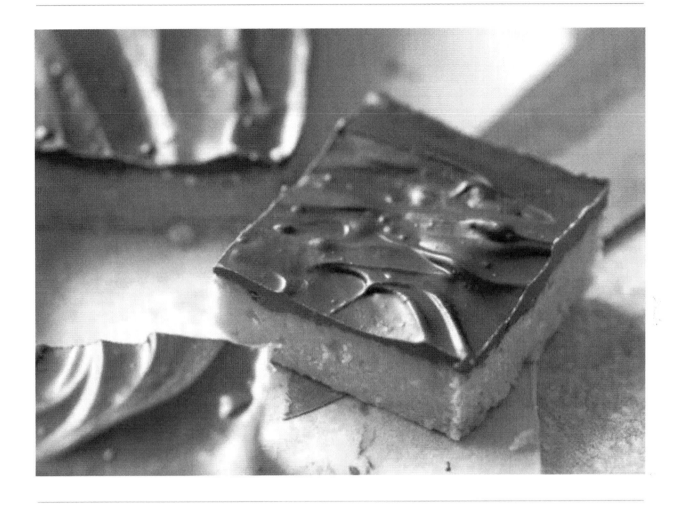

CARBS–17 g   FAT–5 g   PROTEIN–4 g   CALORIES–120

INGREDIENTS

- *2 cups peanut butter*
- *¾ cup flax seed meal*
- *½ cup maple syrup*
- *1 tsp vanilla extract*
- *16 ounces dark chocolate, chopped*

DIRECTIONS

1. Line an 8x8–inch pan with parchment paper and set aside.
2. Melt the peanut butter in a large saucepan. Stir in the vanilla, flaxseed, and syrup. Remove from the heat.
3. Pour into the pan and smooth. Put it in the fridge to rest for a while.
4. Melt the chocolate in a double boiler, stirring continuously with a spatula until it's fully melted and smooth.
5. Pour the chocolate over the peanut butter and smooth it out with spoon.
6. Put in the fridge and let chocolate set completely.
7. Cut into squares and serve.

OATMEAL CHOCOLATE CHIP COOKIES

SERVINGS: 24   PREP TIME: 10 min.   COOK TIME: 20 min.

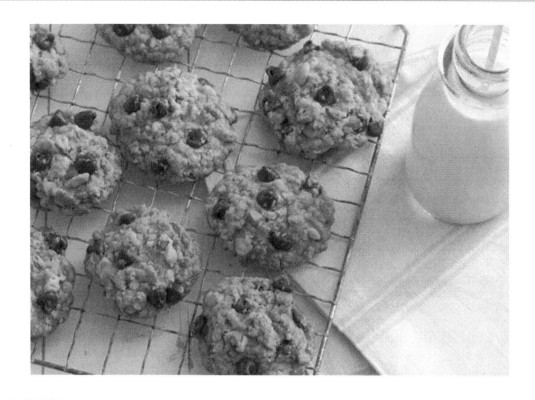

CARBS–18 g   FAT–5 g   PROTEIN–2 g   CALORIES–122

INGREDIENTS

DRY INGREDIENTS:

- 1½ cups rolled oats, lightly pulverized
- 1 cup white whole wheat flour
- ½ tsp baking powder
- 1 tsp ground cinnamon
- Pinch salt

WET INGREDIENTS:

- ½ cup non–salted butter
- 1 cup organic brown sugar, packed
- 1 egg, large
- 1 tsp vanilla extract

FOR THE FINAL DOUGH:

- ½ cup mini chocolate chips

DIRECTIONS

1. Preheat the oven to 350ºF. Line a baking sheet with parchment paper. Set aside.

2. Add the oats to a food processor and blend for 15–20 seconds to shred them into smaller pieces.

3. Add the oats and all of the dry ingredients to a bowl and mix well. Set aside.

4. In another large bowl, mix the butter, sugar, and cream with a hand mixer.

5. Add in the egg and mix. Scrape all of the sides of the bowl, add the vanilla, and mix to make it light and fluffy.

6. Gradually add the dry ingredients to the wet ingredients, continue mixing on a low speed. Fold in the mini chocolate chips.

7. Using a cookie scoop, form dough balls and slightly flatten each of them between your palms. Transfer to a sheet and bake for 10–12 minutes.

8. Remove from the oven and let them cool before serving.

CHOCOLATE CUPCAKES

SERVINGS: 14   PREP TIME: 10 min.   COOK TIME: 20 min.

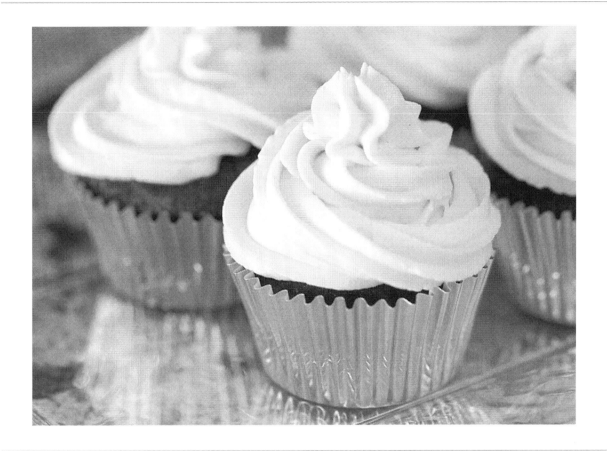

CARBS–18 g   FAT–3 g   PROTEIN–3 g   CALORIES–108

INGREDIENTS

WET INGREDIENTS
- 1 cup unsweetened almond milk
- 1 egg, large
- ¾ cup light brown sugar, packed
- ½ cup nonfat Greek yogurt
- 1 tsp vanilla extract
- 2 Tbsp coconut oil, melted

DRY INGREDIENTS:
- ½ cup all–purpose flour
- ½ cup white whole wheat flour
- ⅓ cup unsweetened dark cocoa powder
- ¾ tsp baking soda
- ½ tsp baking powder

FOR THE FROSTING:
- 1 cup heavy whipping cream
- 2 Tbsp honey

DIRECTIONS

1. Preheat the oven to 350°F.
2. Line a cupcake tin with liners. Spray them with cooking spray.
3. Cream the coconut oil and brown sugar in a bowl with a hand mixer. Add the rest of the wet components and mix until well combined.
4. Mix all of the dry components in another bowl. Then, sift the dry mixture into the wet ingredients, using a sifter.
5. Mix with a hand mixer until smooth, scraping the sides of bowl while mixing.
6. Fill each tin about ⅔–¾ full.
7. Bake for 18–20 minutes.
8. To make the frosting, add the heavy cream and honey to a large bowl.
9. Whip until it starts to form stiff peaks with a hand mixer.
10. Frost right before serving.

CHOCOLATE PEANUT BUTTER MOUSSE

SERVINGS: 1   PREP TIME: 5 min.   COOK TIME: 5 min.

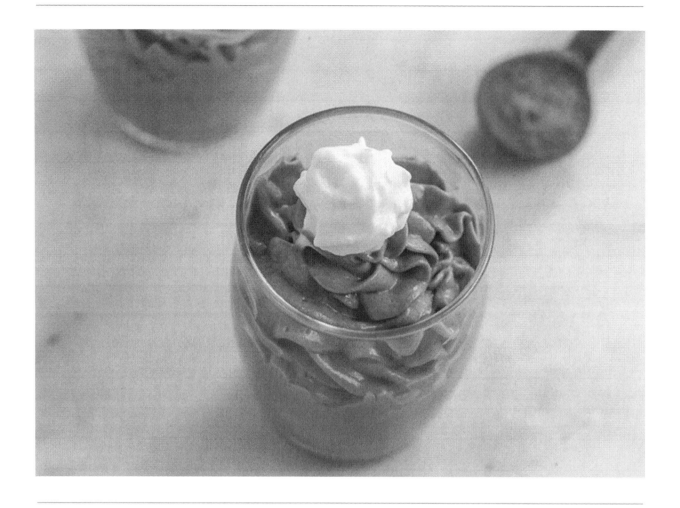

CARBS–19 g   FAT–8 g   PROTEIN–18 g   CALORIES–213

INGREDIENTS

- *⅓ cup vanilla Greek yogurt*
- *1 Tbsp creamy peanut butter*
- *1½ Tbsp cocoa powder*
- *½ cup whipped cream, for serving*

DIRECTIONS

1. Add the peanut butter, yogurt, and cocoa powder in a bowl.
2. Mix until the mixture is well combined.
3. Divide between serving glasses and top with whipped cream.

APPLE PIE BARS

SERVINGS: 12   PREP TIME: 25 min.   COOK TIME: 45 min.

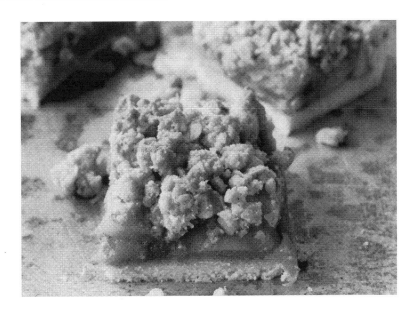

CARBS–41 g   FAT–27 g   PROTEIN–9 g   CALORIES–435

INGREDIENTS

FOR THE CRUST:
- 3 cups superfine almond meal
- 1 cup rolled oats
- 2 Tbsp butter, room temperature
- ¼ cup coconut oil, room temperature
- ¼ cup maple syrup
- 1 tsp vanilla extract
- ⅛ tsp salt
- 1 tsp ground cinnamon
- ¼ tsp ground nutmeg

FOR THE FILLING:
- 6 cups fresh apples, diced
- ¼ cup fresh lemon juice
- ⅔ cup maple syrup
- 1 Tbsp ground cinnamon
- ⅛ tsp salt

FOR THE CRUMBLE TOPPING:
- ⅔ cup rolled oats
- 3 Tbsp butter, room temperature and sliced
- 2 Tbsp brown sugar
- ¼ cup chopped pecans

DIRECTIONS

1. Preheat the oven to 350°F.
2. Line an 8x8–inch baking dish with parchment paper. Set aside.
3. Add all of the ingredients for the crust into a bowl. Mix until it starts to form a crumble and holds its form.
4. Transfer into a baking dish and flatten evenly onto the bottom of the pan.
5. Bake for 15–17 minutes or so until the crumble is golden brown.
6. Meanwhile, add all of the filling ingredients to a pot. Turn to high and let it boil.
7. Switch to low and simmer for 9 minutes, stirring to make the filling thicker.
8. Remove from the heat and mash the apples with a fork.
9. Spread the filling evenly over the crust. Set aside.
10. To prepare the topping, add all of the toppings to a bowl, and cut with a fork until it starts to form a crumble.
11. Spread the crumble topping evenly on top of the filling.
12. Bake for 30 minutes or until the top is golden brown.
13. Take the bars out of oven and let it cool for 10–15 minutes.
14. Put in the fridge for 1 hour before slicing and serve.

FRESH CHERRY CRISP

SERVINGS: 8   PREP TIME: 20 min.   COOK TIME: 30 min.

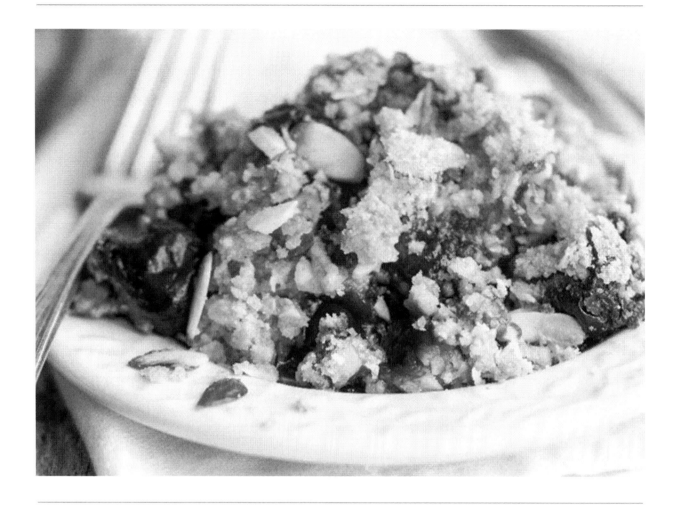

CARBS–42 g   FAT–13 g   PROTEIN–4 g   CALORIES–294

INGREDIENTS

FOR THE FILLING:
- *4 cups pitted cherries, halved*
- *2 Tbsp white whole wheat flour*
- *⅓ cup orange juice*

FOR THE CRISP TOPPING:
- *1½ cups rolled oats*
- *½ cup white whole–wheat flour*
- *½ cup brown sugar*
- *1 tsp cinnamon*
- *⅛ tsp salt*
- *½ cup unsalted butter, softened*

DIRECTIONS

1. Preheat the oven to 375°F.
2. Oil a cake pan with cooking spray.
3. Toss the cherries with flour and orange juice in a bowl. Pour the mixture into the pan and set aside.
4. In another bowl mix all of the crumble components. Cut the butter into the dry ingredients until it starts to form crumbles. Spread the crumble topping evenly over the cherries.
5. Bake until the crumble topping starts to brown (30 minutes).
6. Serve with toppings of your choice.

CHOCOLATE NICE CREAM

SERVINGS: 2   PREP TIME: 20 min.   COOK TIME: 20 min.

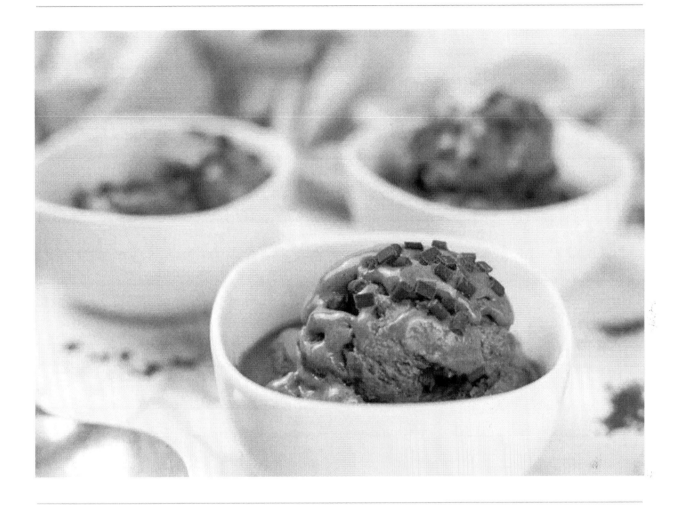

CARBS–39 g   FAT–2 g   PROTEIN–4 g   CALORIES–171

INGREDIENTS

- *2 cups frozen sliced bananas*
- *¼ cup unsweetened cocoa powder*
- *1 tsp vanilla extract*
- *1 Tbsp unsweetened almond milk*
- *1 cup chocolate chips, for serving*

DIRECTIONS

1. Add all of the components to a blender and blend until smooth on high speed.
2. Transfer into a parchment–lined pan. Put into the freezer for 1–2 hours until it has firmed up.
3. Serve with chocolate chips.

FRUIT PIZZA

SERVINGS: 12   PREP TIME: 15 min.   COOK TIME: 20 min.

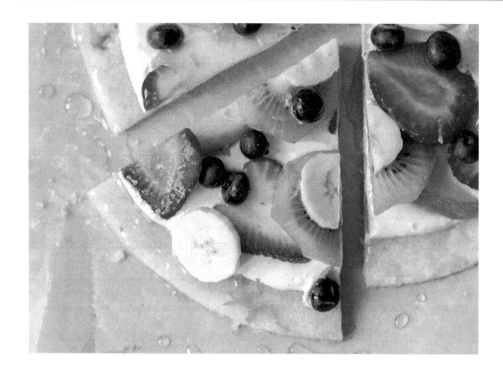

CARBS–18 g   FAT–15 g   PROTEIN–7 g   CALORIES–221

INGREDIENTS

WET INGREDIENTS:
- *1 large egg*
- *1 tsp vanilla extract*
- *¼ cup honey*
- *2 Tbsp coconut oil, softened*

DRY INGREDIENTS:
- *2 cups blanched almond flour*
- *½ cup coconut flour*
- *½ tsp baking soda*
- *Pinch of salt*

FOR THE FILLING:
- *3 oz. cream cheese*
- *½ cup Greek yogurt*
- *1½–2 Tbsp honey*
- *½ orange zest*

FOR THE FRUIT:
- *1½ cups fruit and berries of choice*

DIRECTIONS

1. Preheat the oven to 350°F.
2. Oil a 10–inch round pan with butter. Set aside.
3. Combine all of the wet ingredients in a bowl. Set aside.
4. In another bowl, mix all of the dry components.
5. Gradually stir in the dry ingredients to the wet ones. It will make a thick dough. Mix and knead it with your hands until combined. Form into a ball.
6. Transfer the dough ball into a greased pan and flatten the dough evenly to the bottom.
7. Bake for 15–20 minutes.
8. Meanwhile, add all of the filling ingredients into a blender and blend until creamy.
9. Let the crust cool and remove from the pan. Spread the filling evenly over the crust top.
10. Top the pizza with fruit and berries of your choice and sprinkle with orange zest.
11. It should sit in the fridge for 20 minutes.
12. Cut into pieces and serve.

SPARKLING WATER

SERVINGS: 1 cup   PREP TIME: 10 min.   COOK TIME: 20 min.

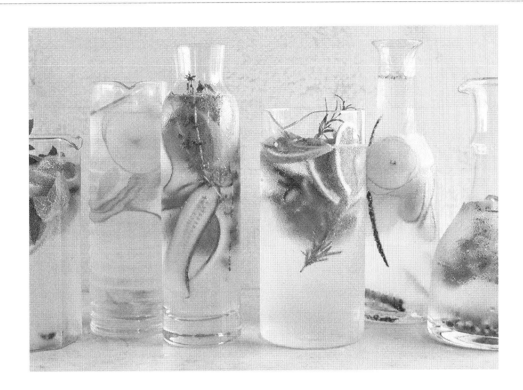

CARBS–3 g   FAT–5 g   PROTEIN–1 g   CALORIES–53

INGREDIENTS

FOR THE BASE:
4 cups sparkling or unsweetened coconut water

GRAPEFRUIT AND STRAWBERRY WATER:
- ½ grapefruit, halved
- 2 thyme sprigs
- ⅓ cup strawberries, sliced
- ½ cup raw ginger, sliced

CUCUMBER AND TANGERINE WATER:
- 5 cucumber slices
- 4 tangerine slices
- 2 thyme sprigs

APPLE AND GINGER WATER:
- 4 Granny Smith apple slices
- 2 (1-inch) lemongrass sticks
- 5 ginger slices

ORANGE AND BASIL WATER:
- 10 grapes, halved
- 3 orange slices
- 6 basil leaves

GREEN TEA WITH MINT AND POMEGRANATE:
- 2 sprigs mint
- 1 bag green tea
- 20 pomegranate seeds, crushed

PEAR AND CINNAMON WATER:
- 1–4 pear slices
- ½ vanilla bean
- 1 cinnamon stick

DIRECTIONS

1. Add your chosen ingredients to the water and put in the fridge overnight to release more flavor.
2. You can remove the rind of the citrus fruit for a less bitter taste, if desired.
3. Pour into glasses and enjoy!

ICED GREEN TEA WITH MINT AND HONEY

SERVINGS: 8   PREP TIME: 2 min.   COOK TIME: 15 min.

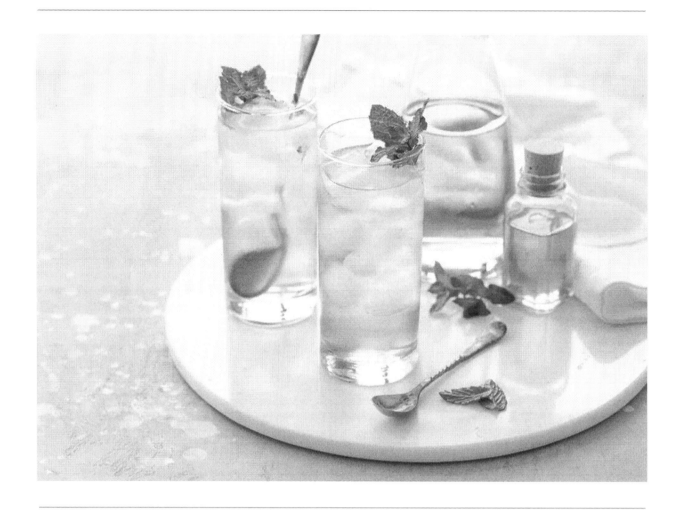

CARBS–8 g   FAT–0 g   PROTEIN–0 g   CALORIES–32

INGREDIENTS

- *4 cups water*
- *4 green tea bags*
- *2 sprigs fresh mint*
- *¼ cup honey*
- *2 cups ice*
- *2 cups cold water*
- *Additional mint sprigs, for serving*
- *Lemon slices, for serving*

DIRECTIONS

1. Pour the water into a saucepan and bring to a boil. Then, turn off the heat and add the tea bags and mint sprigs. Cover and leave for 10 minutes.
2. Discard the tea bags and mint. Add the honey and stir until dissolved.
3. Add the ice, cold water, and tea mixture in a pitcher. Stir until well combined.
4. Let it chill until cold.
5. Serve over ice with a mint sprig.

BLUEBERRY ICED TEA

SERVINGS: 6   PREP TIME: 1 day   COOK TIME: 5 min.

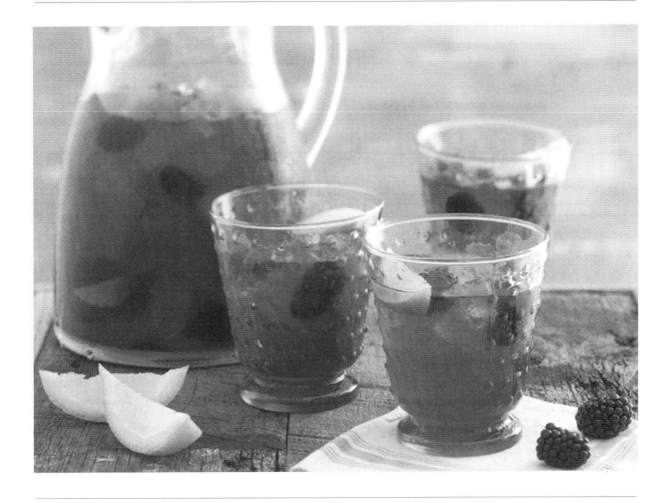

CARBS–10 g   FAT–0 g   PROTEIN–0 g   CALORIES–40

INGREDIENTS

- *2 cups fresh blueberries, more for serving*
- *4 black tea bags*
- *2 cups sugar*
- *1 lemon juice and wedges*
- *7½ cups water*
- *3–4 fresh mint leaves*

DIRECTIONS

1. Add ½ a cup of water and the blueberries to a saucepan over a medium–high heat.
2. Once it is boiling, cook for 3 minutes.
3. Mash the cooked blueberries. Strain the mashed fruit juice into a bowl.
4. Squeeze the blueberry juice into the bowl using the back of a spoon.
5. Pour the blueberry juice, lemon juice, water, and mint leaves into the pitcher.
6. Mix well and add the tea bags. Put in the fridge overnight.
7. Add ice to each glass, then the fresh blueberries, and pour in the blueberry juice.
8. Top with fresh mint leaves and lemon wedges before serving.

ICED BUBBLE MATCHA TEA

SERVINGS: 1   PREP TIME: 5 min.   COOK TIME: 5 min.

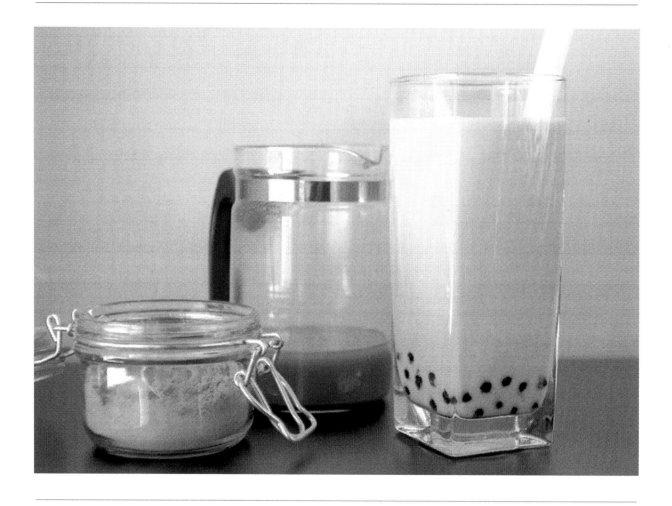

CARBS–53 g   FAT–3 g   PROTEIN–4 g   CALORIES–240

INGREDIENTS

- *1 tsp matcha green tea powder*
- *2 Tbsp hot water*
- *2 Tbsp honey*
- *1 cup almond milk*
- *½ cup ice cubes, more for serving*
- *¼ cup cooked tapioca pearls*

DIRECTIONS

1. Mix the matcha powder with water in a small bowl. Let it brew for 1–2 minutes and set aside.
2. Add the honey, matcha tea, almond milk, and ice into a Vitamix container in this order and lock the lid.
3. Set to Variable 1 and start. Speed up to Variable 10 and blend for 30 seconds.
4. Pour the mixture over the tapioca pearls in a glass and serve.

HONEY MINT LEMONADE

SERVINGS: 7   PREP TIME: 5 min.   COOK TIME: 5 min.

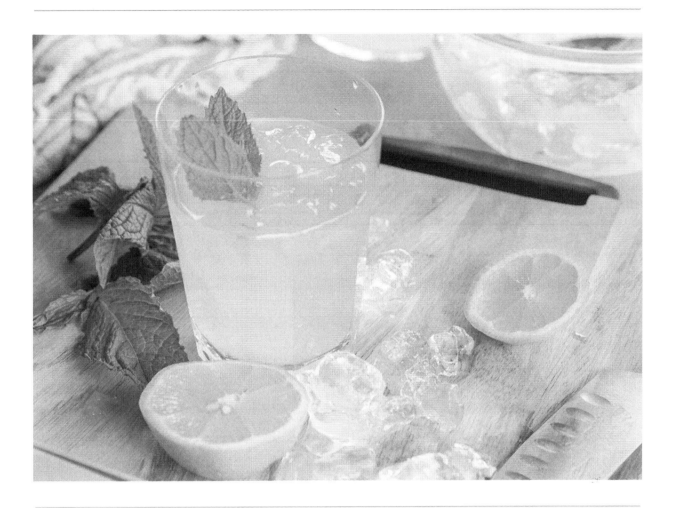

CARBS–23 g   FAT–1 g   PROTEIN–1 g   CALORIES–86

INGREDIENTS

- ½ cup honey
- 1 cup lemon juice
- 1 cup fresh mint leaves
- 6 cups cold water
- Lemon slices and additional mint for garnish

DIRECTIONS

1. Warm 1 cup of water in a small bowl. Add the honey and stir until it has fully dissolved. Add the fresh mint leaves and muddle.
2. Add the rest of the water and lemon juice.
3. Stir until well combined and serve over ice.

STRAWBERRY LEMONADE

SERVINGS: 12   PREP TIME: 5 min.   COOK TIME: 10 min.

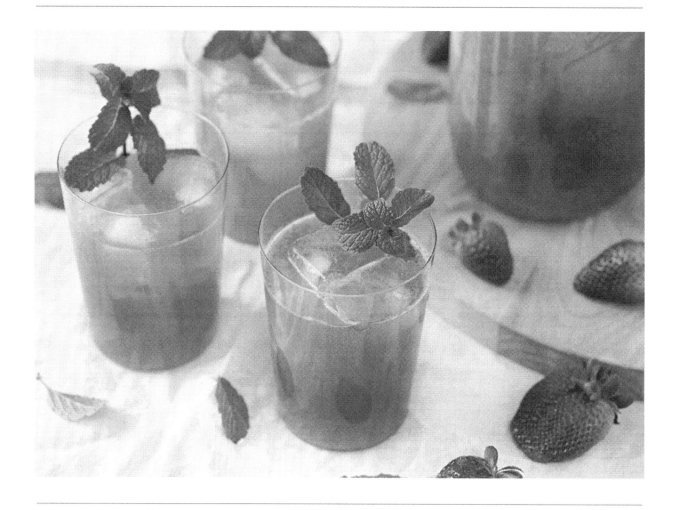

CARBS–23 g   FAT–0 g   PROTEIN–0 g   CALORIES–87

INGREDIENTS

- *8 large strawberries, halved*
- *2 Tbsp white sugar*
- *7 cups water, divided*
- *1 cup white sugar*
- *2 cup lemon juice*
- *Fresh mint leaves, for serving*

DIRECTIONS

1. Add the strawberries to a blender and top with 2 Tbsp sugar. Pour 1 cup of water over the berries. Blend for 1 minute until it's juicy with no chunks.
2. Mix the strawberry juice, 1 cup of sugar, 6 cups of water, and lemon juice in a pitcher. Stir well.
3. Let it chill before serving.
4. Top with fresh mint leaves and enjoy.

HOT CHOCOLATE

SERVINGS: 1   PREP TIME: 5 min.   COOK TIME: 5 min.

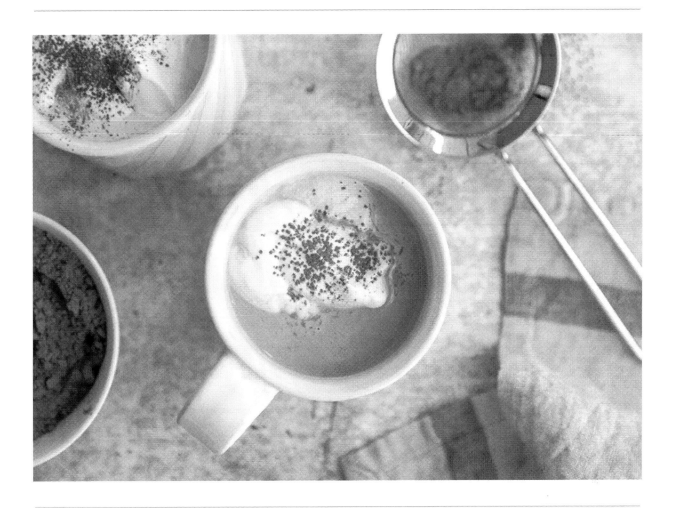

CARBS–17 g   FAT–3 g   PROTEIN–2 g   CALORIES–100

INGREDIENTS

- *1 cup almond milk*
- *1 Tbsp raw cacao powder, more for serving*
- *1 Tbsp pure maple syrup*
- *¼ tsp vanilla extract*
- *Pinch of sea salt*
- *Dairy–free whipped cream, for serving*

DIRECTIONS

1. Mix all of the ingredients (except the cream) in a saucepan over a high heat, whisking to break up clumps.
2. Cook for 3–5 minutes, stirring until smooth and hot. Pour into a cup and serve warm.
3. Top with whipped cream and sprinkle with cacao powder.

LEMON, STRAWBERRY AND BASIL WATER

SERVINGS: 1 cup   PREP TIME: 5 min.   COOK TIME: 5 min.

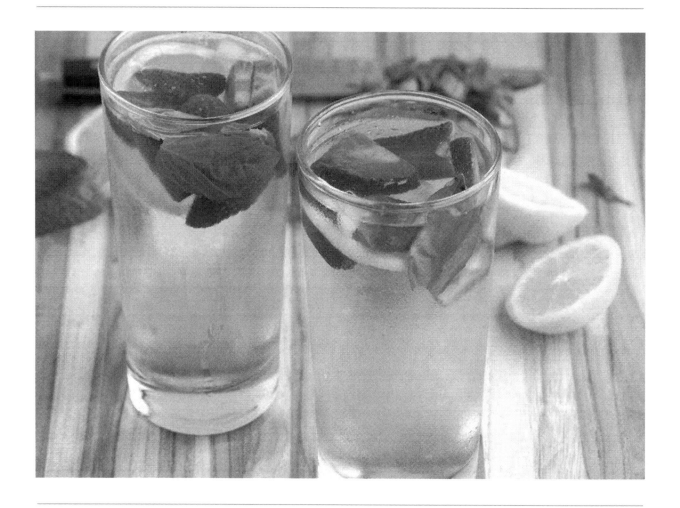

CARBS–3 g   FAT–0 g   PROTEIN–0 g   CALORIES–13

INGREDIENTS

- *1 cup strawberries, hulled and halved*
- *1 lemon juice and slices*
- *1 handful basil leaves, more for serving*
- *3–4 cup filtered water or sparkling water*

DIRECTIONS

1. Add the strawberries and lemon juice to a jar.
2. Scrunch the basil leaves in your hands and slowly stir in with a wooden spoon.
3. Pour the water into the jar, seal and leave for 3–4 hours to infuse.
4. Top the glasses with more basil leaves and a lemon slice before serving.

ELECTROLYTE CITRUS DRINK

SERVINGS: 1   PREP TIME: 5 min.   COOK TIME: 5 min.

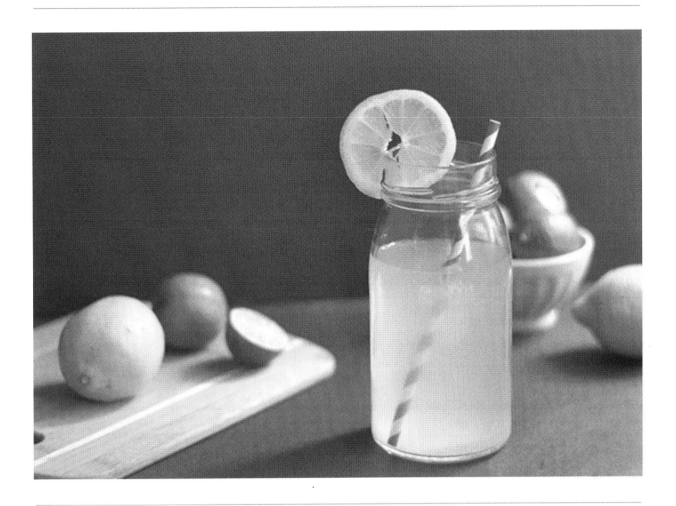

CARBS–17 g   FAT–1 g   PROTEIN–1 g   CALORIES–60

INGREDIENTS

- *1¾ cups herbal tea, water, or coconut water*
- *⅓ tsp pink Himalayan salt*
- *2 tsp raw honey*
- *¼ cup lemon or lime juice*
- *1 tsp calcium/magnesium powder*

DIRECTIONS

1. Brew the tea and let it cool slightly. If using water or coconut water, let it warm slightly.
2. Add the honey, salt, and calcium or magnesium powder. Mix until fully dissolved.
3. Add the juice, then stir well. Taste and adjust the juice or sweetness if needed.
4. Enjoy!

HELP YOUR TEEN TO BE IN HARMONY WITH FOOD

Now that they spend so much more time away from home, it is hard to relinquish control of our kiddos' food. Whether your child is gaining weight as a by–product of puberty or eating out of stress, avoidance, boredom, or just not being as physically active as they used to be is sometimes difficult to tell.

There are many helpful, yet some potentially harmful ways to help your teen feel good about food and their body and it is crucial that you approach this topic in a helpful way.

Teenagers often find themselves in an emotional state with hormones, changes to their body, school stress, and peers... The way you approach body and food image can make or break your relationship with them.

HERE ARE SOME STRATEGIES TO HELP YOUR CHILD FEEL GOOD ABOUT FOOD AND THEIR BODY:

- Avoid panic! Tell your child calmly that you love them, but you have noticed some changes in their eating and exercising habits. Let them know you love them whatever their size or shape, and you're there to help if they want it.
- Help them determine whether changes in food intake and body weight may be associated with puberty, emotional eating, eating more with friends from school, less physical activity because of time limitations or other factors.
- Consider a visit to a doctor for your child to rule out any medical problems.
- Teach your child that body diversity is natural, and that people come in all kinds of shapes and sizes.
- Help your child learn to listen to the internal signals of hunger and fullness in their bodies, rather than focusing on external numbers such as body weight.
- Become a role model for your child's healthy habits and offer to help them work on pleasure exercises and eating because of hunger rather than emotion.

- Help them to develop an outlet for their feelings, such as listening in a non-judgmental manner to their concerns and helping them to work on non–eating coping skills.
- Have family meals when you can and be a role model by eating a wide range of nutritional, satisfying and pleasurable foods
- Store a variety of meal and snack foods in your home, including fruits and vegetables, whole grains, dairy, meat and other proteins, and added satiety fats.
- Have some less nutritious "fun" foods in your pantry, or your child will find them in friends' houses.
- Make your home a comfortable, safe place for your child to talk about their feelings, their changing bodies, and their food intake.

HERE ARE STRATEGIES THAT DON'T HELP:

- DO NOT nag your child or focus on their intake of food. This usually backfires, and your teen may end up eating more as a result.
- DO NOT tell them that some food is "good", and others are "bad."
- DO NOT weigh your child (unless advised by your dietitian or MD on medical grounds).
- DO NOT bribe your child with food as a reward/praise them for not consuming a specific food.
- DO NOT stress the weight of your child by dwelling on any weight loss/weight gain.

In the backdrop of media exposure, diet culture, and the inevitable body comparisons these provide it is so hard for parents these days.

When parents try to restrict the intake of their child's food instead of teaching him/her to listen to hunger and fullness levels, and that all foods can be part of a balanced diet, it usually backfires! Most of the time, children with restricted diets end up eating secretly and eating larger amounts of food than their bodies need, which can result in weight gain and an unhealthy food relationship.

CONCLUSION

Thank you for reading this book and having the patience to try the recipes.

I do hope that you have had as much enjoyment reading and experimenting with the meals as I have had writing the book.

If you would like to leave a comment, you can do so at the Order section–>Digital orders, in your Amazon account.

Stay safe and healthy!

RECIPE INDEX

Dry Weights

OZ		C		
1/2 OZ	1 Tbsp	1/16 C	15 g	
1 OZ	2 Tbsp	1/8 C	28 g	
2 OZ	4 Tbsp	1/4 C	57 g	
3 OZ	6 Tbsp	1/3 C	85 g	
4 OZ	8 Tbsp	1/2 C	115 g	1/4 lb
8 OZ	16 Tbsp	1 C	227 g	1/2 lb
12 OZ	24 Tbsp	1 1/2 C	340 g	3/4 lb
16 OZ	32 Tbsp	2 C	455 g	1 lb

Liquid Conversions

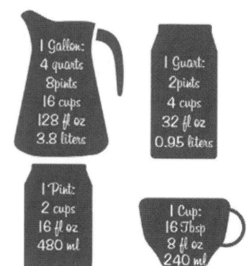

1 Gallon:
4 quarts
8 pints
16 cups
128 fl oz
3.8 liters

1 Quart:
2 pints
4 cups
32 fl oz
0.95 liters

1 Pint:
2 cups
16 fl oz
480 ml

1 Cup:
16 Tbsp
8 fl oz
240 ml

OZ			mL	C	Pt	Qt
1 oz	6 tsp	2 Tbsp	30 ml	1/8 C		
2 oz	12 tsp	4 Tbsp	60 ml	1/4 C		
2 2/3 oz	16 tsp	5 Tbsp	80 ml	1/3 C		
4 oz	24 tsp	8 Tbsp	120 ml	1/2 C		
5 1/3 oz	32 tsp	11 Tbsp	160 ml	2/3 C		
6 oz	36 tsp	12 Tbsp	177 ml	3/4 C		
8 oz	48 tsp	16 Tbsp	237 ml	1 C	1/2 pt	1/4 qt
16 oz	96 tsp	32 Tbsp	480 ml	2 C	1 pt	1/2 qt
32 oz	192 tsp	64 Tbsp	950 ml	4 C	2 pt	1 qt

Fahrenheit to Celcius (F to C)

500 F	= 260 C
475 F	= 245 C
450 F	= 235 C
425 F	= 220 C
400 F	= 205 C
375 F	= 190 C
350 F	= 180 C
325 F	= 160 C
300 F	= 150 C
275 F	= 135 C
250 F	= 120 C
225 F	= 107 C

1 Tbsp: 15 ml

1 tsp: 5 ml

Safe Cooking Meat Temperatures

Minimum temperatures:

USDA Safe at 145 F	USDA Safe at 160 F	USDA Safe at 165 F
Beef Steaks, Briskets, and Roasts; Pork Chops, Roasts, Ribs, Shoulders, and Butts; Lamb Chops, Legs, and Roasts; Fresh Hams, Veal Steaks, Fish, and Shrimp	Ground Meats (except poultry)	Chicken & Turkey, ground or whole

Printed in Great Britain
by Amazon